The COVID-19 Pandemic

Recent Titles in
21st-Century Turning Points

The #MeToo Movement
Laurie Collier Hillstrom

The NFL National Anthem Protests
Margaret Haerens

School Shootings and the Never Again Movement
Laurie Collier Hillstrom

The Vaping Controversy
Laurie Collier Hillstrom

Family Separation and the U.S.–Mexico Border Crisis
Laurie Collier Hillstrom

The College Affordability Crisis
Laurie Collier Hillstrom

The COVID-19 Pandemic

Laurie Collier Hillstrom

21st-Century Turning Points

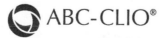

An Imprint of ABC-CLIO, LLC
Santa Barbara, California • Denver, Colorado

Library of Congress Cataloging-in-Publication Data

Names: Hillstrom, Laurie Collier, 1965- author.
Title: The COVID-19 pandemic / Laurie Collier Hillstrom.
Description: Santa Barbara, California : ABC-CLIO, [2021] |
    Series: 21st-century turning points | Includes bibliographical references and index.
Identifiers: LCCN 2020055378 (print) | LCCN 2020055379 (ebook) |
    ISBN 9781440878275 (cloth) | ISBN 9781440878282 (ebook)
Subjects: LCSH: COVID-19 (Disease)—United States.
Classification: LCC RA644.C67 H55 2021 (print) | LCC RA644.C67 (ebook) |
    DDC 362.1962/414—dc23
LC record available at https://lccn.loc.gov/2020055378
LC ebook record available at https://lccn.loc.gov/2020055379

ISBN: 978-1-4408-7827-5 (print)
       978-1-4408-7828-2 (ebook)

25 24 23 22 21   1 2 3 4 5

This book is also available as an eBook.

ABC-CLIO
An Imprint of ABC-CLIO, LLC

ABC-CLIO, LLC
147 Castilian Drive
Santa Barbara, California 93117
www.abc-clio.com

This book is printed on acid-free paper ∞

Manufactured in the United States of America

Contents

Series Foreword

21st-Century Turning Points is a general reference series that has been crafted for use by high school and undergraduate students as well as members of the general public. The purpose of the series is to give readers a clear, authoritative, and unbiased understanding of major fast-breaking events, movements, people, and issues that are transforming American life, culture, and politics in this turbulent new century. Each volume constitutes a one-stop resource for learning about a single issue or event currently dominating America's news headlines and political discussions—issues or events that, in many cases, are also driving national debate about our country's leaders, institutions, values, and priorities.

Each volume in the *21st-Century Turning Points* series begins with an **Overview** of the event or issue that is the subject of the book. It then provides a suite of informative chronologically arranged narrative entries on specific **Landmarks** in the evolution of the event or issue in question. This section provides both vital historical context and insights into present-day news events to give readers a full and clear understanding of how current issues and controversies evolved.

The next section of the book is devoted to examining the **Impacts** of the event or issue in question on various aspects of American life, including political, economic, cultural, and interpersonal implications. It is followed by a chapter of biographical **Profiles** that summarize the life experiences and personal beliefs of prominent individuals associated with the event or issue in question.

Finally, each book concludes with a topically organized **Further Resources** list of important and informative resources—from influential books to fascinating websites—to which readers can turn for additional information, and a carefully compiled subject **Index**.

These complementary elements, found in every book in the series, work together to create an evenhanded, authoritative, and user-friendly tool for gaining a deeper and more accurate understanding of the fast-changing nation in which we live—and the issues and moments that define us as we move deeper into the twenty-first century.

CHAPTER ONE

Overview of the COVID-19 Pandemic

The pandemic that engulfed the world in 2020 is the type of rare historic event that defines the collective memories and experiences of everyone alive to witness it. It started when a previously unknown type of coronavirus, SARS-CoV-2, made the leap from animals to humans through zoonotic transfer. Doctors in China first identified the new pathogen in December 2019, when they began seeing clusters of patients with COVID-19, the severe respiratory illness it caused. Ease of transmission from person to person through airborne droplets, combined with global interconnectedness via air travel and supply chains, facilitated the spread of the deadly virus around the world. "We are living in the perfect storm right now," said Anthony Fauci, director of the U.S. National Center for Allergy and Infectious Diseases (Kuchler 2020). By November 2020—less than a year from its emergence—the coronavirus had infected 55 million people and caused 1.3 million deaths worldwide. The United States accounted for the highest number of confirmed COVID-19 cases, at 11 million, as well as the most deaths, at 250,000.

The pandemic fundamentally altered so many aspects of modern life that a generation of people will forever view their experiences through the lens of "before COVID" and "after COVID." Protective face masks became a reflexive addition to everyday apparel—stashed in pockets, purses, backpacks, and cars—as well as a contentious political issue. "Lockdown" joined the vernacular, as cities and states issued stay-at-home orders, closed nonessential businesses, and restricted social gatherings and discretionary travel. Prolonged school closures disrupted learning and development for 50 million children across the United States. Twenty million Americans lost their jobs, and millions more made the transition to working remotely. Airline travel ground to a virtual halt, sporting and cultural events were canceled, city streets stood quiet and empty, and stores ran out of toilet paper and hand sanitizer. "In just a few months, COVID-19 has forced billions of people, in nearly every country on earth, into a panicked withdrawal from society," Michael Specter wrote in the *New Yorker* (2020).

The U.S. Pandemic Response

Although the sudden emergence of COVID-19 caught most of the world off guard, scientists have long warned about the possibility of an infectious disease pandemic. Earlier pandemics killed millions of people and altered the course of human history, so some experts argued it was only a matter of time before a new pathogen threatened humanity. "We live in evolutionary competition with microbes—bacteria and viruses," Nobel Prize–winning biologist Joshua Lederberg said as early as 1990. "There is no guarantee that we will be the survivors" (Specter 2020). Despite what many considered close calls with outbreaks of Severe Acute Respiratory Syndrome (SARS), Ebola virus disease, and H1N1 influenza in the twenty-first century, few nations placed a high priority on pandemic preparedness. In 2018, for instance, U.S. President Donald Trump disbanded a directorate-level office within the National Security Council (NSC) dedicated to global health security and biodefense. Critics argued that this change eliminated a source of federal government expertise in the area of pandemic readiness.

After the first COVID-19 cases appeared in China, the coronavirus quickly spread through Asia and into Europe. The United States confirmed its first case on January 20, 2020, in a man from Washington State with a history of travel to China. Two days later, when a reporter asked Trump if he felt concerned about the potential for a global pandemic, he replied, "No, not at all. We have it totally under control. It's one person coming in from China, and we have it under control. It's going to be just fine" (Leonhardt 2020). Although the president suspended travel to the United States from China on January 31, he continued to minimize the threat posed by COVID-19 in public statements throughout the month of February. He falsely claimed the disease was no worse than the seasonal flu, asserted without evidence that the coronavirus would disappear with the arrival of warmer weather, and described warnings of an approaching pandemic as a Democratic "hoax" intended to sink the U.S. economy and harm his reelection campaign. Meanwhile, in a private conversation with reporter Bob Woodward in February, Trump acknowledged that he intentionally downplayed the seriousness of the situation. "I wanted to always play it down," he stated. "I still like playing it down, because I don't want to create a panic" (Friedersdorf 2020).

Critics claimed that the Trump administration wasted weeks that it could have spent preparing the nation for the impending public health crisis. "Mitigation required leadership," said *Slate* writer William Saletan (2020). "The president needed to tell Americans that the crisis was urgent and that life had to change. Instead, he told them everything was fine." As the coronavirus invaded country after country, public health experts emphasized the importance of conducting tests to identify and isolate carriers of SARS-CoV-2—some of whom never developed symptoms—and to guide the deployment of personnel and resources to contain outbreaks. U.S. testing programs became mired in delays, glitches, supply shortages, and political wrangling, however, while Trump administration officials repeatedly denied that a problem existed. "Anybody that needs a test gets a test," Trump (2020) declared on March 6. While the president bragged about the relatively low number of COVID-19 cases in the United States compared to other countries, public health officials warned that the lack of testing was allowing the virus to spread undetected.

By the time the World Health Organization (WHO) declared COVID-19 a global pandemic on March 11, the United States had recorded more than 1,000 cases in 36 states. On March 16, Trump began appearing at the daily televised press briefings held by the White House Coronavirus Task Force—a panel he had convened six weeks earlier to provide the American people with up-to-date information about COVID-19. After downplaying the severity of the crisis for nearly two months, the president acknowledged the need to slow the spread of the virus. Trump urged the American people to cancel gatherings of more than ten people, avoid crowded bars and restaurants, work from home if possible, move classes online, and self-quarantine at home if they experienced symptoms. "With several weeks of focused action, we can turn the corner and turn it quickly," he declared (McCaskill, Kenen, and Cancryn 2020).

As the task force briefings went on, however, critics charged that Trump's daily appearances did little to inform or reassure the public. Rather than focusing on the COVID-19 pandemic, the president often used the platform to praise his administration's performance, attack his political opponents, engage in verbal sparring with reporters, and tout signs of a quick economic recovery. In addition, Trump frequently provided misinformation that contradicted the advice of medical experts. He repeatedly promoted the antimalaria drug hydroxychloroquine as a potential cure before it had been tested, for instance, and he once made the dangerous suggestion that COVID-19 patients consume or inject disinfectants. Trump also refused to wear a face mask in accordance with public health recommendations, which encouraged some of his followers to eschew mask wearing as a political statement.

In the absence of a coordinated, nationwide pandemic response, state governors, city mayors, and local public health officials implemented a hodgepodge of measures to combat the spread of the coronavirus. California became the first state to issue a mandatory stay-at-home order on March 19, and most other states enacted similar restrictions over the next week. The state lockdowns—which typically involved closing schools and nonessential businesses, banning social events and discretionary travel, and requiring residents to remain at home except to buy food or access health care—created challenges and hardships for millions of Americans. The U.S. unemployment rate skyrocketed from an 80-year low of 3.5 percent in February to 14.7 percent in April. Consumer spending plummeted, causing many stores and restaurants to go out of business. School closures and a lack of day care options forced many parents to juggle the competing demands of online learning, childcare, and working from home. Individuals grappled with depression, substance abuse, and other mental health issues stemming from isolation, fear, and uncertainty.

The U.S. Congress responded to the mounting economic crisis by passing the Coronavirus Aid, Relief, and Economic Security (CARES) Act, which Trump signed into law on March 27. At $2.2 trillion, the CARES Act became the largest economic stimulus package ever enacted in U.S. history. The legislation allocated $300 billion to provide one-time economic impact payments to more than 160 million Americans in an effort to strengthen the social safety net and prevent families from descending into poverty during the pandemic. In addition, the CARES Act provided more than $500 billion in interest-free loans, tax breaks, and emergency aid for large corporations, as well as more than $350 billion in forgivable loans for small businesses through the Paycheck Protection Program (PPP). Finally, the CARES Act provided $340 billion to help state and local governments respond to the public health crisis, as well as $150 billion to aid hospitals and health care facilities in treating COVID-19 patients.

Despite the widespread implementation of mitigation measures, the number of COVID-19 cases in the United States increased exponentially in late March and April. The nation reached 500,000 cases on April 11 and 1 million—or around one-third of the world's total cases—on April 28.

The massive influx of patients exceeded the capacity of hospitals in some hard-hit areas, prompting governors to plead for federal assistance in acquiring personal protective equipment (PPE), constructing temporary hospitals to increase bed capacity, and contracting with American industries to produce ventilators. Trump responded by claiming that the states had everything they should need, blaming the governors for mishandling the crisis, and dismissing the complaints as politically motivated.

Tensions rose in late April and May as Trump increasingly asserted his authority and pressured governors to lift stay-at-home orders and reopen their states. He argued that the lockdowns devastated the U.S. economy and disrupted the daily lives of Americans without significantly reducing the spread of SARS-CoV-2. A growing number of citizens expressed frustration, anger, and resentment at being forced to hunker down and shelter in place for weeks on end. Some opponents characterized the government-imposed restrictions as unconstitutional infringements on their individual rights and freedoms. When anti-lockdown protests erupted in two dozen states in late April, Trump encouraged the demonstrators to "liberate" their states. Critics charged that the president's message weakened citizens' commitment to following social-distancing measures and undermined the shared sense of national responsibility and sacrifice necessary to combat the coronavirus.

The stay-at-home orders and other mitigation measures proved effective in reducing daily COVID-19 cases to manageable levels in much of the country. Many states—especially those led by Republican governors in the South and Southwest—responded by relaxing or eliminating restrictions in late April and early May. Arizona, Florida, Georgia, South Carolina, Texas, and other states that reopened early showed signs of economic recovery, marked by increases in consumer spending and decreases in unemployment. By June, however, they also experienced a resurgence in coronavirus cases. Nationwide, the number of confirmed cases surged above 75,000 per day in July—twice as high as the peak daily rates in mid-April—prompting some public health officials to declare a second wave underway.

Politicization of a Public Health Crisis

According to public health experts, mounting an effective response to the coronavirus required the United States to develop a coordinated national strategy and enlist the support of the American people in implementing it. "Coping with a pandemic is one of the most complex challenges a society can face. To minimize death and damage, leaders and citizens must orchestrate a huge array of different resources and tools," James Fallows wrote in the *Atlantic* (2020). "It is a challenge that the United States did not meet." Instead, the U.S. pandemic response was severely hampered by political polarization, entrenched partisan loyalties, distrust of government, skepticism of science, staunch individualism, and widespread misinformation. "You can't promote public health without social solidarity. Here is a case where it's clear that our fate is linked to the fate of our neighbors," New York University sociologist Eric Klinenberg explained. "Physical distancing and isolation only work if people respect the order and take heed of the scientific facts" (Friedman 2020).

Politics and partisanship played a major role in determining state and federal COVID-19 policies, such as stay-at-home orders and timelines for economic reopening. Partisan affiliation also affected the degree of public compliance with such recommendations as mask wearing and social distancing, with Democrats overwhelmingly supporting these measures and Republicans—following Trump's example—largely opposing them. Combined with misinformation spread through media outlets and social media, critics charged that political polarization undermined the U.S. coronavirus response at the expense of the nation's public and economic health. As scientists gathered new evidence about the transmission of SARS-CoV-2, for instance, the U.S. Centers for Disease Control and Prevention (CDC) revised its earlier recommendations and urged citizens to wear masks. Opponents of mask wearing took advantage of this reversal to cast doubt on the CDC's credibility and justify their own position. "We're kind of building the airplane as we fly it and we need to be able to change course when we get new evidence," said infectious disease expert Samuel Scarpino. "But it becomes harder to have those conversations and get buy-in from the public as the whole process becomes more politicized" (Thomson-DeVeaux 2020).

As president during the pandemic, Trump bore much of the responsibility for the nation's lack of preparedness and ineffective response. Critics pointed to his denial of the severity of the crisis, his emphasis on reopening the economy despite the public health risks, his propensity for spreading false or misleading information, and his personal disregard for such basic precautions as mask wearing and social distancing as detrimental factors in his performance. "With our lives upended by a disease that by the end of his term will have led to the deaths of well more than a quarter-million Americans, we naturally judge the president by his handling of the pandemic," wrote Jerry Adler of Yahoo! News (2020), "and the verdict on his stewardship is clear: It was a disaster characterized by wishful thinking; scientific illiteracy; and inconsistent, dishonest, and reckless policymaking." As national case rates surpassed 100,000 per day in the autumn months, Trump's insistence on holding large, in-person campaign rallies and White House events resulted in him contracting COVID-19.

Negative assessments of Trump's handling of the pandemic contributed to the end of his presidency, as voters elected Democratic candidate Joe Biden in the November 2020 presidential election. Biden offered a seven-point plan for defeating COVID-19 that included mandating mask usage nationwide, expanding testing capacity, providing federal guidance to states and local communities, addressing racial health disparities, and investing in the development of treatments and vaccines. Pandemic-weary Americans received a long-awaited piece of good news shortly after the election, when the CDC announced that several different vaccines had proven up to 95 percent effective in preventing new coronavirus infections. Public health experts predicted that these vaccines could end the COVID-19 pandemic in the United States by the spring of 2021. "The tasks that lie ahead—manufacturing vaccines at scale, distributing them . . . , and persuading wary Americans to take them—are not trivial, but they are all within the realm of human knowledge," Sarah Zhang wrote in the *Atlantic* (2020). "The most tenuous moment is over: The scientific uncertainty at the heart of COVID-19 vaccines is resolved. Vaccines work. And for that, we can breathe a collective sigh of relief."

Further Reading

Adler, Jerry. 2020. "How Will History View Trump—And Us?" Yahoo! News, November 7, 2020. https://news.yahoo.com/how-will-history-view-trump-and-us-193258976.html.

Fallows, James. 2020. "The Three Weeks That Changed Everything." *Atlantic,* June 29, 2020. https://www.theatlantic.com/politics/archive/2020/06/how-white-house-coronavirus-response-went-wrong/613591/.

Fidler, David P. 2020. "Coronavirus: A Twenty-Year Failure." Think Global Health, March 23, 2020. https://www.thinkglobalhealth.org/article/coronavirus-twenty-year-failure.

Friedersdorf, Conor. 2020. "Trump Failed the 3 A.M. Test." *Atlantic,* October 11, 2020. https://www.theatlantic.com/ideas/archive/2020/10/trump-failed-3-am-test/616678/.

Kuchler, Hannah. 2020. "Anthony Fauci: 'We Are Living in the Perfect Storm.'" *Financial Times,* July 10, 2020. https://www.ft.com/content/57834c2c-a078-4736-9173-8fb32cfbbf4e.

Leonhardt, David. 2020. "A Complete List of Trump's Attempts to Play Down Coronavirus." *New York Times,* March 15, 2020. https://www.nytimes.com/2020/03/15/opinion/trump-coronavirus.html.

McCaskill, Nolan D., Joanne Kenen, and Adam Cancryn. 2020. "'This Is a Very Bad One': Trump Issues New Guidelines to Stem Coronavirus Spread." Politico, March 16, 2020. https://www.politico.com/news/2020/03/16 /trump-recommends-avoiding-gatherings-of-more-than-10-people -132323.

Saletan, William. 2020. "The Trump Pandemic." Slate, August 9, 2020. https:// slate.com/news-and-politics/2020/08/trump-coronavirus-deaths -timeline.html.

Specter, Michael. 2020. "How Anthony Fauci Became America's Doctor." *New Yorker,* April 10, 2020. https://www.newyorker.com/magazine/2020/04 /20/how-anthony-fauci-became-americas-doctor.

Thomson-DeVeaux, Amelia. 2020. "Republicans and Democrats See COVID-19 Very Differently. Is That Making People Sick?" FiveThirtyEight.com, July 23, 2020. https://fivethirtyeight.com/features/republicans-and-demo crats-see-covid-19-very-differently-is-that-making-people-sick/.

Trump, Donald. 2020. "Remarks by President Trump after Tour of the Centers for Disease Control and Prevention, Atlanta, Georgia." The White House, March 7, 2020. https://www.whitehouse.gov/briefings-statements/remarks -president-trump-tour-centers-disease-control-prevention-atlanta-ga/.

Zhang, Sarah. 2020. "The End of the Pandemic Is Now in Sight." *Atlantic,* November 18, 2020. https://www.theatlantic.com/health/archive/2020 /11/vaccines-end-covid-19-pandemic-sight/617141/.

CHAPTER TWO

Landmark Events in the COVID-19 Pandemic

This chapter explores important milestones and events in the COVID-19 pandemic and U.S. efforts to contain it. It reviews infectious disease outbreaks that changed human history, examines elements of modern life that made the world vulnerable to pathogens, and discusses U.S. and international pandemic preparedness efforts. It then explores the emergence of the novel coronavirus SARS-CoV-2 in China and tracks its global spread during the spring of 2020. Finally, the chapter analyzes the often competing response measures enacted by the Trump administration and the governors of individual states to prevent transmission of COVID-19 and limit the pandemic's economic and social impacts.

Disease Epidemics and Pandemics in History (1350–2014)

Humans have been susceptible to infectious diseases caused by microorganisms—such as bacteria, viruses, protozoa, and parasites—throughout recorded history. As humans shifted away from nomadic, hunter-gatherer lifestyles toward living in communities and building civilizations, their proximity allowed disease outbreaks to spread from person to person and cause epidemics. As improvements in travel, trade, and transport forged links between humans occupying distant parts of the world, these connections allowed disease outbreaks to spread beyond national or regional boundaries to become pandemics.

At many points, epidemics or pandemics of such diseases as bubonic plague, cholera, influenza, leprosy, malaria, polio, smallpox, tuberculosis, and yellow fever have altered human history. Around 1350, for instance, a bubonic plague pandemic swept through Asia and Europe, killing an estimated 100 million people, or about one-third of the world's total population. Historians have attributed both the collapse of the British feudal system and the advent of the Italian Renaissance to the so-called Black Death. Beginning in 1492, Spanish explorers carried such diseases as influenza, measles, and smallpox on their journeys to North America and the Caribbean. These unfamiliar germs caused epidemics that killed approximately 56 million people, or around 90 percent of the indigenous population, which precipitated the downfall of the Aztec civilization in Mexico and the European colonization of the New World.

By the twentieth century, Louis Pasteur and other scientists had developed the germ theory of disease and identified the pathogens responsible for several deadly diseases. These discoveries led to a greater understanding of communicability and to improvements in sanitation practices and preventative measures. During the 1918 Spanish flu pandemic, for instance, government officials in many countries closed schools and businesses and ordered citizens to remain indoors or wear face masks in public. These measures proved to be no match for what turned out to be one of the deadliest pandemics in history, which killed between 20 and 50 million people as it swept across Europe to the United States, often carried by troops fighting in World War I. The flu pandemic exacerbated wartime shortages of medical personnel, overwhelmed hospitals and funeral parlors, and disrupted food production and basic services.

The twentieth century also saw the development of vaccines that reduced the incidence of many infectious diseases, eliminated others from certain countries or regions, and eradicated smallpox worldwide by 1980. Nevertheless, new pathogens continued to appear, including some that infected humans through contact with an animal host—a process called zoonotic transfer. The human immunodeficiency virus (HIV), for instance, originated in West Africa among monkeys and chimpanzees and eventually infected humans who prepared or consumed the animals as bushmeat. Left untreated, HIV causes Acquired Immune Deficiency Syndrome (AIDS), which destroys the immune system and leaves people vulnerable to rare cancers and secondary infections.

In the United States, AIDS first appeared in otherwise healthy gay men in San Francisco and New York City in 1981. During the early years of the ensuing public health crisis, the misconception that HIV spread through casual contact led to a surge in hostility and discrimination toward LGBT people. Researchers later learned that the virus was only transmitted through the direct exchange of bodily fluids, such as blood, semen, or breast milk. AIDS grew into a global pandemic, killing an estimated 700,000 people in the United States and 35 million around the world. Although doctors developed diagnostic tests to identify carriers of HIV and antiretroviral drugs to prevent them from developing AIDS, the virus continues to infect an estimated 1.8 million new people every year (Levine 2019).

From SARS to MERS

Despite humankind's long history of fighting epidemics, the first significant outbreak of the twenty-first century caught many nations off guard and raised concerns about the world's preparedness for the next global pandemic. Severe Acute Respiratory Syndrome (SARS) originated in November 2002 in Guangdong Province, China, where a cluster of patients exhibited a highly contagious, atypical form of pneumonia that did not respond to treatment. Their symptoms included difficulty breathing, dry cough, fever, and head and body aches.

Doctors initially suspected avian influenza, which infected several other patients in China at that time. Researchers later identified SARS as a coronavirus, part of a large family of viruses characterized by spiky projections that resemble the points of a crown ("corona" in Latin). Some coronaviruses primarily infect birds or nonhuman mammals, while the four varieties previously known to infect humans typically caused mild symptoms associated with the common cold. Scientists determined horseshoe bats to be the original host species of SARS, and they traced the initial human exposure to palm civets—raccoon-like creatures sold in live-animal markets and consumed as delicacies in China.

The Chinese Ministry of Health did not report the situation to the World Health Organization (WHO) until mid-February 2003, by which time the country had recorded 300 cases and 5 deaths. A 2004 report criticized China's response to the outbreak, claiming it had been hindered by a "fatal period of hesitation regarding information sharing and action." China also hid facts about the disease outbreak from the public, according to the report, which led to "heightened anxieties, fear, and widespread speculation" (Radcliffe 2020).

Although WHO officials immediately alerted the Global Outbreak Alert and Response Network (GOARN)—which consists of national health organizations, academic institutions, and technical experts from around the world—the SARS virus had already spread outside of China. A Chinese doctor who developed respiratory symptoms after treating SARS patients traveled to Hong Kong, where he transmitted the virus to at least 16 other international travelers in his hotel before he became severely ill, checked into a hospital, and died ten days later. "A global outbreak was thus seeded from a single person on a single day on a single floor of a Hong Kong hotel," wrote a team of analysts from GOARN (Mackenzie et al. 2004).

SARS quickly spread to 26 other countries. The virus infected 8,096 people and caused 774 deaths before it was contained in July 2003 through international collaboration and an aggressive public health response. Many experts considered the SARS outbreak a close call and said the situation could have easily spiraled out of control to cause a global pandemic. "Nobody really predicted that SARS would not continue to be a problem," said epidemiologist Arnold S. Monto. "But by public health measures—including isolation and proper precautions—it was possible to put the genie back in the bottle" (Radcliffe 2020).

In the aftermath of SARS, many scientists and public health experts urged governments around the world to develop comprehensive plans to respond to future disease outbreaks. They warned that such factors as climate change, mass displacement and migration, international travel and tourism, and global commerce created countless new opportunities for the transmission of infectious diseases. "It was only a matter of time before one of those diseases proved truly catastrophic. The world could avert the worst consequences if it started planning," noted an editorial in the *New York Times*. "But SARS was quickly contained (in part because the virus itself was so deadly that it was easy to detect). The disease faded from public consciousness and, with it, any sense of urgency over future outbreaks" (Editorial Board 2020).

The United States recorded only eight laboratory-confirmed cases of SARS during the 2003 outbreak—all of them among people who had traveled to affected areas in Asia—and no deaths. As a result, public health authorities proved unable to convince the federal government to dedicate significant resources toward preparing for a future coronavirus outbreak. Instead, much of the U.S. infectious disease response in the early 2000s focused on the threat of bioterrorism and involved stockpiling vaccines for weaponized anthrax and smallpox. "One of the paradoxes of preparedness is that you have to constantly prepare for something that might or might not happen, and you might well prepare for the wrong thing," sociologist Andrew Lakoff explained. "It's highly likely that you won't be ready for what actually unfolds" (Lewis 2020).

The next global pandemic emerged in the United States in April 2009. The H1N1 influenza virus, also known as swine flu, originated on hog farms in Mexico, infected humans through zoonotic transmission, and quickly spread around the world. Over the next year, it affected more than 60 million people and caused between 151,000 and 575,000 deaths, including nearly 12,500 in the United States. Unlike seasonal influenza, which usually takes the greatest toll on people older than 65, the H1N1 pandemic mainly affected children and young adults who lacked immunity from exposure to similar viruses. The age factor, combined with existing knowledge of flu vaccines, gave it a relatively low mortality rate and helped mitigate public fears about transmission. Although President Barack Obama declared a national public health emergency and initiated some preparedness efforts, the Great Recession resulted in $900 million in budget cuts for health security programs between 2010 and 2011 (Diamond 2020).

In 2012, another coronavirus emerged in Saudi Arabia that caused an outbreak of a new disease called Middle East respiratory syndrome (MERS). Scientists again traced the virus to bats and learned that humans became exposed through contact with infected camels. Although MERS exhibited a high mortality rate of 35 percent, it rarely spread outside of hospitals because human-to-human transmission occurred through close, sustained contact. MERS affected around 2,500 people worldwide, mostly in the Arabian Peninsula and South Korea, with only two cases reported in the United States.

Pandemic Preparedness

In 2014, an epidemic of Ebola virus disease (EVD) in West Africa generated some movement toward preparing for the possibility of a global infectious disease pandemic. EVD is a form of hemorrhagic fever that causes fever, headache, muscle aches, skin rash, vomiting, diarrhea, loss of liver and kidney function, and severe internal and external bleeding. The disease can be caused by several species of Ebola viruses, which originated in nonhuman primates and spread to humans through contact with infected animals during the preparation and consumption of bushmeat. Africa experienced two dozen Ebola outbreaks in the four decades since scientists first identified the virus in 1976. The 2014 epidemic was the largest one, involving more than 28,600 cases and 11,300 deaths. Although Ebola can only be transmitted through direct contact with the bodily fluids of an infected person or animal, the disease's gruesome progression and 50 percent mortality rate generated a great deal of public apprehension.

Americans called for action after a man from Liberia with EVD sought treatment at an emergency room in Dallas, Texas. After initially being misdiagnosed and sent home, the man returned to the hospital when his symptoms worsened and died two weeks later. Although he transmitted the disease to two nurses involved in his care, both recovered. The presence of Ebola in the United States served as a wake-up call for public health officials. The Obama administration treated it as a national security issue and requested $6 billion in emergency funding to put measures in place to protect the American people and to help contain the outbreak at its source. The administration sent 3,000 civilian and military personnel to Africa to establish treatment centers and provide medical assistance and scientific expertise. It also funded research toward vaccine development and the purchase of personal protective equipment (PPE) for hospitals.

In a December 2014 speech to researchers at the National Institutes of Health (NIH), Obama emphasized the importance of preparing for infectious disease outbreaks. "We were lucky with H1N1—that it did not prove to be more deadly. We can't say we're lucky with Ebola because obviously it's having a devastating effect in West Africa, but it is not airborne in its transmission," he stated. "There may and likely will come a time in which we have both an airborne disease that is deadly. And in order for us to deal with that effectively, we have to put in place an infrastructure—not just here at home, but globally—that allows us to see it quickly, isolate it quickly, respond to it quickly. . . . It is a smart investment for us to make. It's not just insurance; it is knowing that down the road we're going to continue to have problems like this—particularly in a globalized world where you move from one side of the world to the other in a day" (Obama 2014).

Infectious disease experts recommended a number of measures be put in place to prevent a future outbreak from spreading to become a global pandemic. They suggested training hospital personnel in the most effective techniques of infection control, for instance, and creating a national stockpile of PPE to ease supply disruptions in an emergency. Experts also recommended increasing funding for state public health departments, which played a vital role in pandemic response by disseminating public information, conducting diagnostic tests, tracing contacts with infected persons, establishing quarantines, and collecting data. Likewise, they suggested fully funding federal health agencies, such as the NIH and the Centers for Disease Control and Prevention (CDC), to support research and development of diagnostic tests, treatments, vaccines, and disease monitoring systems. Finally, infectious disease experts recommended that the U.S. government support developing nations in their efforts to contain the spread of pathogens. "The best strategy," according to the *New*

York Times editorial, "is to help other nations—wherever they are—fight humanity's common enemy over there before we have to fight it over here" (Editorial Board 2020).

The Global Health Security (GHS) Index examined the level of preparedness for epidemics and pandemics in all 195 countries around the world. Each nation received a score between 0 and 100 based on six factors relating to infectious disease control: prevention, detection, rapid response, health system capability, compliance with international standards, and risk level. The average score for all countries came out at a dismal 40.2. Although the United States ranked number one based on its high income, stable government, and effective health care system, it still only achieved a score of 83.5. The rest of the top five nations by GHS Index score included the United Kingdom (77.9), the Netherlands (75.6), Australia (75.5), and Canada (75.3) (LePan 2020).

Further Reading

Diamond, Dan. 2020. "Inside America's Two-Decade Failure to Prepare for Coronavirus." Politico, April 11, 2020. https://www.politico.com/news/magazine/2020/04/11/america-two-decade-failure-prepare-coronavirus-179574.

Editorial Board. 2020. "Here Comes the Coronavirus Pandemic." *New York Times,* February 29, 2020. https://www.nytimes.com/2020/02/29/opinion/sunday/corona-virus-usa.html.

Lakoff, Andrew. 2017. *Unprepared: Global Health in the Time of Emergency.* Berkeley: University of California Press.

LePan, Nicholas. 2020. "Ranked: Global Pandemic Preparedness by Country." Visual Capitalist, March 20, 2020. https://www.visualcapitalist.com/global-pandemic-preparedness-ranked/.

Levine, David. 2019. "HIV Statistics: What Are the Current Numbers?" *U.S. News and World Report,* September 10, 2019. https://health.usnews.com/conditions/hiv-aids/articles/hiv-statistics.

Lewis, Wayne. 2020. "Disaster Response Expert Explains Why U.S. Wasn't More Prepared for the Pandemic." USC Dornsife, March 24, 2020. https://dornsife.usc.edu/news/stories/3182/why-u-s-wasnt-better-prepared-for-the-coronavirus/.

Mackenzie, J. S., P. Drury, A. Ellis, T. Grein, K. C. Leitmeyer, S. Mardel, A. Merianos, B. Olowokure, C. Roth, R. Slattery, G. Thomson, D. Werker, and M. Ryan. 2004. "The WHO Response to SARS and Preparations for the Future." In *Learning from SARS: Preparing for the Next Disease Outbreak,* edited by Stacey Knobler, Adel Mahmoud, Stanley Lemon, Alison Mack, Laura Sivitz, and Katherine Oberholtzer Washington, DC: National Academies Press, 2004. https://www.ncbi.nlm.nih.gov/books/NBK92476/.

Obama, Barack. 2014. "Remarks by the President on Research for Potential Ebola
    Vaccines." The White House, December 2, 2014. https://obamawhitehouse
    .archives.gov/the-press-office/2014/12/02/remarks-president-research
    -potential-ebola-vaccines.
Radcliffe, Shawn. 2020. "Can We Learn Anything from the SARS Outbreak to
    Fight COVID-19?" Healthline, March 11, 2020. https://www.healthline
    .com/health-news/has-anything-changed-since-the-2003-sars-outbreak.

A Novel Coronavirus Emerges in China (2019)

In late 2019, a mysterious illness appeared in China that would test global preparedness for an infectious disease pandemic. A cluster of patients in Wuhan—the bustling capital city of Hubei Province in Central China, with a population of more than 11 million—developed viral pneumonia with symptoms resembling those exhibited by SARS patients in 2003. By the time Chinese health authorities reported the outbreak to the World Health Organization (WHO) on December 31, there were 27 confirmed cases. Scientists soon identified the pathogen as a new or novel type of coronavirus that previously had not been known to infect humans. They named the virus SARS-CoV-2 and the disease it caused COVID-19 (short for "coronavirus disease 2019"). The highly communicable virus spread quickly, and on March 11, 2020, WHO officially declared it a global pandemic. By early June, at least 6.5 million people around the world had contracted COVID-19 and nearly 388,000 had died from it ("Coronavirus World Map" 2020).

Wuhan Experiences a Disease Outbreak

Doctors in Wuhan first began seeing patients with SARS-like symptoms—such as fever, cough, difficulty breathing, chest congestion, headache, muscle aches, fatigue, and loss of taste or smell—in mid-December 2019. They initially described the mysterious ailment as "viral pneumonia of unknown cause." Further investigations showed that two-thirds of these early patients had visited the Huanan Seafood Wholesale Market, a so-called "wet market" where vendors in open-air stalls sold fresh meat and produce, as well as many different species of live wild animals to be slaughtered for food or traditional medicine or kept as exotic pets. Scientists noted that these markets provided ideal conditions for the zoonotic transfer of pathogens. "When you bring animals together in these unnatural situations, you have the risk of human diseases emerging," said disease ecologist Kevin Olival. "If the animals are housed in bad conditions under a lot of stress, it might create a better opportunity for them to shed virus and to be sick" (Akpan 2020).

Around December 24, Wuhan Central Hospital began sending samples of lung fluid from the atypical pneumonia patients to laboratories for testing. When the reports came back a few days later, most identified the pathogen responsible as a novel, previously unknown coronavirus. Doctors initially assumed that the patients had contracted this virus through direct contact with infected animals at the wet market, and they doubted whether human-to-human transmission had occurred. One sample, however, erroneously showed a positive result for SARS. Alarmed at the potential for a new SARS epidemic, the director of Wuhan Central Hospital's emergency department, Ai Fen, took a photograph of the report and sent it to a colleague at a nearby hospital on December 27. The photo circulated quickly among the city's medical professionals, as they warned each other to take appropriate precautions in case they were facing a SARS outbreak.

Later that evening, Wuhan Central Hospital administrators admonished Ai for disclosing information about the mysterious disease prematurely. She received a reprimand from the hospital's disciplinary committee for "spreading rumors" and "harming stability" (Kuo 2020). Administrators did not allow Ai to alert her staff in the emergency department to the potential danger. Another doctor who shared information about the emerging virus on social media, ophthalmologist Li Wenliang, ended up being detained by Wuhan police. The authorities released him only after he signed a statement admitting to "making false comments" that had "seriously disrupted [the] social order" (Yu 2020). Eight other doctors received punishments as well.

Chinese officials claimed that they curtailed the doctors' warning messages because they wanted to prevent the release of incorrect information that might cause widespread public panic. Critics charged that this secretiveness prevented the medical community from adopting protective measures and allowed the virus to spread. The Chinese Centre for Disease Control and Prevention continued to insist that the virus came from animals, for instance, even as hospitals began seeing patients with no connection to the wet market. "We watched more and more patients come in as the radius of the spread of infection became larger," Ai recalled. "I knew there must be human to human transmission" (Kuo 2020).

On December 31, the Wuhan Municipal Health Commission issued the first public announcement about the outbreak of atypical pneumonia. Health officials confirmed 27 cases and recommended that citizens wear face masks in public, even though they still denied having any evidence of human-to-human transmission. The Chinese National Health Commission also notified WHO, which dispatched a rapid response team to investigate. A WHO spokesman downplayed the severity of the situation, however, and expressed doubt that the illness was related to SARS. "There are many potential causes of viral pneumonia, many of which are more common than severe acute respiratory syndrome coronavirus," the spokesman said. "WHO is closely monitoring this event and will share more details as we have them" ("China Pneumonia Outbreak" 2020).

On January 7, Chinese scientists successfully isolated and identified the virus responsible for the disease outbreak. Genetic sequencing revealed it to be a novel coronavirus, around 75 percent related to the SARS virus and up to 96 percent identical to a known bat coronavirus called RATG13, suggesting that it had a zoonotic origin. They named the new coronavirus SARS-CoV-2 and the disease it caused COVID-19. Within a few days, Chinese authorities shared genetic information about SARS-CoV-2 with health agencies and scientific research centers around the world to aid in the development of diagnostic tests, treatments, and vaccines. Experts noted that it only took about a month from the first appearance of COVID-19 in humans for scientists to identify the virus, compared to around five months for SARS. "Having information quickly really helps public health officials start to contain it," said epidemiologist Anne W. Rimoin. "The ability to rapidly identify viruses—and identify that you have a new virus—is an extraordinary and important new development" (Radcliffe 2020).

China Imposes a Strict Lockdown

On January 11, Chinese media reported the death of a 61-year-old man who had been a frequent customer at the Wuhan wet market. He became the first confirmed death associated with complications from COVID-19. The number of cases had doubled every week since the beginning of the outbreak, and by mid-January the virus spread beyond Wuhan to infect people in other Chinese provinces. On January 20, the Chinese National Health Commission finally confirmed that SARS-CoV-2 could be spread through human-to-human transmission.

By this time, according to WHO's first situation report, the novel coronavirus had also begun to spread outside of China, with confirmed cases in Japan, South Korea, Thailand, and the United States. The American patient, a man in his thirties, had recently returned to Washington State following a trip to Wuhan. The head of the Chinese Communist Party, Xi Jinping, issued the government's first public statement about the outbreak that day. He urged citizens to avoid unnecessary travel, practice social distancing, and wear face masks in public. He also told government officials to "put people's lives and health first" and to "release epidemic information in a timely manner and deepen international co-operation" (Belluz 2020).

On January 23, Chinese authorities introduced extraordinary public health measures intended to contain the COVID-19 outbreak. At this point, Wuhan had recorded more than 500 cases and 17 deaths. The government notified residents that the city would be subject to a complete lockdown, quarantine, or *cordon sanitaire* ("sanitary barrier") beginning at 10:00 a.m. that day. Officials announced that all public transportation—including airplanes, buses, ferries, subways, and trains—would be suspended to restrict travel into, out of, or within Wuhan. In addition, Chinese authorities shut down highways and banned the use of private vehicles in the city. "The lockdown of 11 million people is unprecedented in public health history," said Gauden Galea, a WHO representative in China. Although the strict quarantine went beyond WHO guidelines, he called it "a very important indication of the commitment to contain the epidemic in the place where it is most concentrated" (Crossley 2020).

Over the next few days, the Chinese government extended the travel restrictions to include 12 other cities in Hubei Province, containing a total of around 50 million residents. Officials also closed schools, universities, and museums, instituted remote-work rules for most businesses, and required people to remain at home except to buy food or medicine. In the meantime, hospitals in Wuhan and the surrounding area struggled to cope with growing numbers of COVID-19 cases. Chinese authorities constructed several emergency field hospitals and converted convention centers and other facilities into temporary hospitals to help treat patients.

The lockdown came as the nation prepared to celebrate the Chinese New Year, a major holiday that typically coincided with the peak travel season in China, with upwards of 350 million people taking vacations or visiting family members. Some critics questioned the severity of the restrictions, arguing that they infringed on individual rights. Others expressed doubts as to whether the quarantine would be effective in containing the spread of the virus. In addition, some observers worried that the lockdown would force healthy people to remain in close quarters with sick ones and prevent food and medical supplies from reaching affected areas.

China's aggressive response to the coronavirus spurred the international community to take action. On January 27, the U.S. Centers for Disease Control and Prevention (CDC) issued an advisory recommending that Americans avoid all nonessential travel to China. In addition, the CDC established screening procedures to check travelers arriving from China for symptoms of COVID-19. Many other countries put travel restrictions in place over the next few days, and dozens of international airlines canceled all flights to and from China. On January 30, WHO formally designated the SARS-CoV-2 outbreak as a Public Health Emergency of International Concern, meaning that the risk had spread beyond national borders and warranted an immediate, coordinated international response. By this time, China had recorded more than 7,700 confirmed cases of COVID-19 and 170 deaths, and the virus had spread outside of China to affect at least 82 people in 18 other countries (WHO 2020).

Delays and Secrecy Hamper International Response

Over the next several weeks, as China expanded the lockdowns to cover nearly half of its total population of 1.4 billion, observers around the world watched anxiously to gauge the effectiveness of the response. Public health researchers found that the travel bans and control measures significantly slowed the spread of the coronavirus in China. Although China recorded 80,000 cases of COVID-19 between December and March, a model simulation by University of Southampton emerging-disease experts Lai Shengjie and Andrew Tatum estimated that the number of cases could have reached 8 million without any restrictions. If Chinese authorities had acted three weeks earlier, however, and limited contact between citizens at the beginning of January, Shengjie and Tatum estimated that they could have reduced the total number of cases to around 4,000 and potentially prevented a global pandemic. "The delay of China to act is probably responsible for this world event," said University of Michigan public health researcher Howard Markel (Cyranoski 2020).

In the early stages of the outbreak, Chinese authorities silenced whistle-blowers who attempted to alert the public and repeatedly denied the possibility of human-to-human transmission. Critics charged that this reluctance to share information cost Dr. Li Wenliang his life. Li contracted the virus by treating infected patients at Wuhan Central Hospital and died of complications from it on February 7, 2020, at age 34. "If the officials had disclosed information about the epidemic earlier I think it would have been a lot better," Li told reporters shortly before his death. "There should be more openness and transparency" (Yu 2020). Li's death led to an outpouring of grief and anger among Chinese citizens, as well as to public demands for less government suppression of information and censorship of individual speech.

As the coronavirus spread around the world in early 2020, scientists worked to uncover the source of the initial outbreak. Experts at the Wuhan Institute of Virology (WIV) raised doubts about the theory that

SARS-CoV-2 made the jump from animals to humans at the Wuhan wet market. They took tissue samples from all of the animals sold at the market and found no evidence of infection. "I haven't seen anything that makes me feel, as a researcher who studies zoonotic disease, that this market is a likely option," said Georgetown University scientist Colin Carlson (Letzter 2020). Instead, experts concluded that an already infected human must have transmitted the virus to other customers at the market directly.

Questions about the origins of the virus, coupled with concerns about China's secrecy, fueled conspiracy theories that SARS-CoV-2 may have been intentionally created as a biological weapon or accidentally released from the WIV or another laboratory. U.S. Secretary of State Mike Pompeo accused China of covering up details about the source of the virus, claiming that the information was "in the possession of only the Chinese Communist Party" (Brennan and Schick 2020). Pompeo also said he had "enormous evidence" that the virus originated in a Chinese lab, although he never revealed that evidence publicly and investigations by U.S. intelligence agencies concluded that SARS-CoV-2 was naturally occurring rather than "man-made or genetically modified" (Brennan and Schick 2020).

U.S. President Donald Trump also criticized the Chinese government's handling of the COVID-19 crisis and unwillingness to cooperate with the international community. When Dr. Shi Zhengli, a specialist in bat coronaviruses at the WIV, reported that SARS-CoV-2 shared genetic similarities with the RATG13 virus found in horseshoe bats, for instance, Trump expressed skepticism. "They talk about a certain kind of bat, but that bat wasn't in that area," he said of the Wuhan market where some of the first cases appeared. "That bat wasn't sold at that wet zone. It wasn't sold there. That bat is 40 miles away. So a lot of strange things are happening, but there is a lot of investigation going on and we're going to find out" (Brennan and Schick 2020).

Based on its high rate of human-to-human transmissibility—which often indicates that a virus has adapted to survive in a particular host species—epidemiologists speculated that the virus may have been circulating in humans for months before the Wuhan outbreak brought it to medical attention. "How long it took to adapt to human populations, and under what circumstances that happened, is harder to say," said Chris Beyrer, a public health expert from Johns Hopkins University. "Could it be that there was a bat-to-human transmission somewhere else, and it just turned out that the density of this industrial city of Wuhan is where the eruption first appeared? That is theoretically possible" (Brennan and Schick 2020). Some scientists noted that Chinese workers could have been exposed to a bat coronavirus by processing bat carcasses or collecting guano for use in traditional medicines. Alternatively, the bats could have infected an intermediate species, such as widely trafficked pangolins, that later infected humans.

In the interest of identifying the source of the virus, the U.S. government demanded that the Chinese Ministry of Health grant access for investigators to check stored samples at Chinese blood banks for antibodies to SARS-CoV-2. Political tensions and travel restrictions made collaboration difficult, however, and Chinese authorities declined offers of assistance from WHO representatives, U.S. officials, and academic researchers from other countries. "They continue to be opaque and they continue to deny access for this important information that our researchers, our epidemiologists need," Pompeo stated (Brennan and Schick 2020). On March 24, Chinese Premier Li Keqiang announced that the coronavirus outbreak had been successfully contained in China. As the number of COVID-19 cases increased around the world, Chinese authorities imposed strict new measures to prevent reintroduction of the virus, including a mandatory 14-day quarantine for international travelers.

Further Reading

Akpan, Nsikan. 2020. "New Coronavirus Can Spread between Humans, but It Started in a Wildlife Market." *National Geographic,* January 21, 2020. https://www.nationalgeographic.com/science/2020/01/new-coronavirus -spreading-between-humans-how-it-started/.

Belluz, Julia. 2020. "Did China Downplay the Coronavirus Outbreak Early On?" *Vox,* January 27, 2020. https://www.vox.com/2020/1/27/21082354/corona virus-outbreak-wuhan-china-early-on-lancet.

Brennan, Margaret, and Camilla Schick. 2020. "Finding Coronavirus' Patient Zero; and a Guilty Bat." CBS News, May 7, 2020. https://www.cbsnews .com/news/coronavirus-patient-zero-bat-index-case/.

"China Pneumonia Outbreak: Mystery Virus Probed in Wuhan." BBC News, January 3, 2020. https://www.bbc.com/news/world-asia-china-50984025.

"Coronavirus World Map." 2020. *Guardian,* June 4, 2020. https://www.the guardian.com/world/2020/jun/04/coronavirus-world-map-which -countries-have-the-most-covid-19-cases-and-deaths.

Crossley, Gabriel. 2020. "Wuhan Lockdown 'Unprecedented,' Shows Commitment to Contain Virus: Who Representative in China." Reuters, January 23, 2020. https://www.reuters.com/article/us-china-health-who-idU SKBN1ZM1G9.

Cyranoski, David. 2020. "What China's Coronavirus Response Can Teach the Rest of the World." *Nature,* March 17, 2020. https://www.nature.com /articles/d41586-020-00741-x.

Kuo, Lily. 2020. "Coronavirus: Wuhan Doctor Speaks Out against Authorities." *Guardian,* March 11, 2020. https://www.theguardian.com/world/2020/mar/11/coronavirus-wuhan-doctor-ai-fen-speaks-out-against-authorities.

Letzter, Rafi. 2020. "The Coronavirus Didn't Really Start at That Wuhan 'Wet Market.'" LiveScience, May 28, 2020. https://www.livescience.com/covid-19-did-not-start-at-wuhan-wet-market.html.

Ma, Josephine. 2020. "Coronavirus: China's First COVID-19 Case Traced Back to November 17." *South China Morning Post,* March 13, 2020. https://www.scmp.com/news/china/society/article/3074991/coronavirus-chinas-first-confirmed-covid-19-case-traced-back.

Radcliffe, Shawn. 2020. "Can We Learn Anything from the SARS Outbreak to Fight COVID-19?" Healthline, March 11, 2020. https://www.healthline.com/health-news/has-anything-changed-since-the-2003-sars-outbreak.

World Health Organization. 2020. "Novel Coronavirus (2019-nCoV) Situation Report—10." January 30, 2020. https://www.who.int/docs/default-source/coronaviruse/situation-reports/20200130-sitrep-10-ncov.pdf?sfvrsn=d0b2e480_2.

Yu, Verna. 2020. "'Hero Who Told the Truth': Chinese Rage over Coronavirus Death of Whistleblower Doctor." *Guardian,* February 7, 2020. https://www.theguardian.com/global-development/2020/feb/07/coronavirus-chinese-rage-death-whistleblower-doctor-li-wenliang.

COVID-19 Reaches the United States (January 20–March 10, 2020)

Three weeks after China reported the Wuhan COVID-19 outbreak to the World Health Organization (WHO), the first confirmed case emerged in the United States. Although the U.S. Centers for Disease Control and Prevention (CDC) began conducting health screenings of airline passengers arriving from Wuhan on January 17, 2020, the initial patient had returned home to Washington State two days earlier. Upon developing symptoms that matched those listed in a CDC health bulletin, the man went to a hospital, where he tested positive for the SARS-CoV-2 virus on January 20. That same day, Chinese scientists and WHO officials said conclusively for the first time that the virus could be spread through human-to-human transmission.

On January 22—as Chinese authorities prepared to impose a total lockdown of Wuhan's 11 million residents to contain the outbreak—a reporter asked President Donald Trump if he felt concerned about the potential for a global pandemic. "No, not at all," he replied. "We have it totally under control. It's one person coming in from China, and we have it under control. It's going to be just fine" (Leonhardt 2020). According to critics, this response marked the beginning of a seven-week period in which Trump ignored warnings from medical experts, downplayed the severity of COVID-19, promoted conspiracy theories and fake cures, and failed to prepare the nation for the impending public health crisis. By early November, the United States had documented more than 10 million confirmed cases and nearly 250,000 deaths in the coronavirus pandemic. "Trump's attempts to downplay the crisis, along with his declarations of success and confusing U-turns, have produced a disaster for the country," wrote CNN correspondent Frida Ghitis (2020).

A Traveler Tests Positive

After Chinese health authorities reported the COVID-19 outbreak to WHO on December 31, 2019, the CDC began preparing for the coronavirus to make its way to the United States. On January 8, for instance, the CDC issued a public health alert to doctors across the country, warning them to look out for patients with respiratory symptoms and a history of travel to China. CDC experts also worked to develop diagnostic tests to confirm the presence of SARS-CoV-2 and treatment guidelines for patients who tested positive. On January 17, the CDC introduced public health screening measures for passengers arriving from Wuhan at three major U.S. airports, in Los Angeles, New York City, and San Francisco. Finally, the CDC activated its Emergency Operations Center to assist state and local health authorities in containing the virus.

These measures did not prevent a 35-year-old man from returning home to Snohomish County, Washington—north of Seattle—on January 15 following a trip to visit family members in Wuhan, China. The man did not go to the live-animal market where the outbreak seemed to be centered, and he did not knowingly come into contact with anyone who appeared to be ill. After developing a fever and cough, however, the man recognized his symptoms in a CDC health bulletin and decided to seek medical attention. He reported to a local urgent care center, where tests for influenza, rhinovirus, and other common pathogens came back negative. Based on the patient's symptoms and travel history, doctors then conducted a nasal-swab test for the coronavirus and sent it to the CDC laboratory. When the results came back positive on January 20, the CDC Emergency Operations Center immediately notified the state and local public health departments.

Health officials decided to transfer the patient to Providence Regional Medical Center in Everett, Washington. They transported him in a mobile isolation unit and placed him in a biohazard chamber used to quarantine patients with infectious diseases. Doctors and nurses involved in his treatment either interacted with him remotely over a video system or wore full protective equipment, including respirator helmets with face shields, when making physical contact. They mainly monitored his vital signs, provided supportive care, and managed his symptoms for the first few days. After five days in the hospital, the patient developed pneumonia and was placed on oxygen. At this point, CDC experts recommended an experimental antiviral medication called remdesivir that had been used to treat the Ebola virus. The patient began showing improvement the next day, and he felt well enough to be released from the hospital in early February. In the meantime, state and local public health investigators traced the man's contacts to determine whether he may have transmitted the virus to other people.

The second travel-related case of COVID-19 in the United States appeared on January 24, when a woman developed symptoms after having returned to Chicago on January 13 from a visit to Wuhan. This patient accounted for the first confirmed local transmission of the virus within the United States, as her husband also tested positive for SARS-CoV-2 on January 30. It later became clear, however, that the virus had probably reached the United States several weeks before the first confirmed cases appeared. A 57-year-old woman from Santa Clara County, California, died on February 6 from what tissue samples later revealed to be complications from COVID-19. She apparently became infected through community spread of the virus in early January, prior to the first reported U.S. case. Since she had no recent history of travel to China, doctors did not initially test for the coronavirus and instead attributed her death to a heart attack. After the COVID-19 connection became clear, Santa Clara County health officials reclassified the deaths of several other people as being caused by the pandemic.

Warnings and Preparations

In the early stages of the COVID-19 crisis, President Trump and other administration officials asserted that no one viewed an infectious disease outbreak as an imminent threat to national security. They claimed that they could not have been expected to prepare for a scenario that they never anticipated occurring. "Nobody knew there'd be a pandemic or an epidemic of this proportion," Trump stated. "Nobody has ever seen anything like this before" (Rieder 2020). Many scientists, public health experts, and intelligence officials contradicted this claim and insisted that they had warned world leaders for years about the need to prepare for such an eventuality. "Anybody who knows national security, anybody who knows global health, knows development issues, understood that we were not only inevitably going to face another global pandemic, but in fact, that the world was overdue," said Susan Rice, former national security adviser to President Barack Obama (Capehart 2020).

In 2012, for instance, the RAND Corporation global policy think tank issued a risk assessment report that described pandemics as "an existential threat, capable of destroying America's way of life," as well as "a real possibility in the here and now" (Rieder 2020). Shortly before Trump took office in 2017, Obama administration officials discussed the potential for disease outbreaks in a national security briefing and shared a 69-page "playbook" outlining key pandemic response strategies. "We included a pandemic scenario because I believed then, and I have warned since, that emerging infectious disease was likely to pose one of the gravest risks for the new administration," said Lisa Monaco, Obama's former homeland security adviser (Rieder 2020). In 2019, the U.S. intelligence community emphasized the importance of pandemic preparedness in its annual *Worldwide Threat Assessment* report. "The United States and the world will remain vulnerable to the next flu pandemic or large-scale outbreak of a contagious disease that could lead to massive rates of death and disability, severely affect the world economy, strain international resources, and increase calls on the United States for support," the report warned (Rieder 2020).

Critics claimed that the Trump administration reduced the nation's pandemic preparedness by disbanding a directorate-level office within the National Security Council (NSC) dedicated to global health security and biodefense. The Obama administration established this office in 2014 in response to an Ebola outbreak. Trump's third national security adviser, John Bolton, eliminated it as a standalone unit during a 2018 reorganization of the NSC and folded it into another unit focused on counterproliferation and biodefense. Critics argued that this change prompted several experts to leave the NSC and shifted the group's area of emphasis and expertise from pandemics involving naturally occurring pathogens to terrorist attacks involving manmade biological weapons. When reporters asked Trump whether the reorganization had hampered the administration's response to the coronavirus, the president reiterated his view of the pandemic as an unforeseeable event. "You never really know when something like this is going to strike and what it's going to be," he stated (Trump 2020). Later, Trump responded to questions about the pandemic preparedness office by claiming not to know about it or denying that it had been disbanded.

After the CDC confirmed the first COVID-19 case in the United States on January 20, it took more than a week for the Trump administration to establish the White House Coronavirus Task Force, under the leadership of Secretary of Health and Human Services Alex Azar, to oversee national efforts to prevent the spread of the virus. On January 30, the day WHO designated the coronavirus outbreak as a Public Health Emergency of International Concern and warned countries to prepare, Trump told supporters that "We have it very well under control. We have very little problem in this country at this moment—five. And those people are all recuperating successfully" (Leonhardt 2020).

The following day, administration officials announced travel restrictions that prohibited foreign citizens from entering the United States if they had traveled to China in the previous two weeks. Some experts praised the move, arguing that it could prevent travelers from carrying SARS-CoV-2 into the country and give the government more time to plot containment strategies. White House spokesman Hogan Gidley called the travel restrictions a "bold, decisive action which medical professionals say will prove to have saved countless lives" (Eder et al. 2020). By the time the restrictions took effect on February 2, however, a *New York Times* analysis estimated that 380,000 passengers had already flown to the United States directly from China since the beginning of the COVID-19 outbreak, including 4,000 from Wuhan. In addition, because the restrictions did not apply to American citizens or their immediate family members, another 40,000 people arrived from China in the two months after they took effect (Eder et al. 2020).

Trump Downplays the Threat

Critics contended that the Trump administration could have done more to prepare the nation's medical system to treat an influx of COVID-19 patients, such as developing rapid-result diagnostic testing capability, acquiring personal protective equipment (PPE) and distributing it to hospitals, increasing bed capacity through the construction of temporary hospitals, and contracting with American industries to produce ventilators. Two physicians who served in the Trump administration—Luciana Borio, former director of medical and biodefense preparedness at the NSC, and Scott Gottlieb, former commissioner of the Food and Drug Administration (FDA)—urged the president to adopt such measures in a January 28 *Wall Street Journal* article entitled "Act Now to Prevent an American Epidemic." "If public-health authorities don't interrupt the spread soon, the virus could infect many thousands more around the globe, disrupt air travel, overwhelm health care systems, and, worst of all, claim more lives," they wrote. "The good news: There's still an opening to prevent a grim outcome. . . . But authorities can't act quickly without a test that can diagnose the condition rapidly" (Borio and Gottlieb 2020).

Public health experts noted that widespread testing would allow them to track the spread of the virus, deploy personnel and resources to treat it, and determine the best strategies to contain it. Testing and early detection grew even more vital when scientists learned that infected people could transmit SARS-CoV-2 even if they did not experience symptoms. Although the CDC began sending test kits to public health laboratories in affected areas on February 5, the initial tests had technical problems that affected their reliability. The issue remained unresolved on February 24, when the Association of Public Health Laboratories pleaded for more test kits. "We are now many weeks into the response with still no diagnostic or surveillance test available outside of the CDC for the vast majority of our member laboratories," the group wrote. Two days later, Trump told reporters that "We're testing everybody that we need to test. And we're finding very little problem" (Gilson, Thompson, and Jeffery 2020).

Critics charged that the Trump administration could have purchased functional tests from WHO or relaxed FDA regulations to allow hospitals, research institutions, and private laboratories to develop their own tests. Instead, administration officials repeatedly denied that a problem existed. "Anybody that needs a test gets a test," Trump (2020) declared on March 6. "They're there. They have the tests. And the tests are beautiful." In reality, the limited availability of tests forced public health officials to reserve them for symptomatic patients with known exposure or a history of travel to affected areas. Although the lack of testing initially kept the number of U.S. cases low relative to other countries, critics charged that it allowed SARS-CoV-2 to spread undetected. "We just twiddled our thumbs as the coronavirus waltzed in," said Harvard University epidemiologist William Hanage (Leonhardt 2020).

As COVID-19 cases increased, Trump often minimized the severity of the disease by comparing it to the seasonal flu and claiming that the virus would go away on its own. "I think it's going to work out fine," he told an interviewer on February 19. "I think when we get into April, in the warmer weather, that has a very negative effect on that and that type of a virus." A week later, Trump told a crowd that the coronavirus was "going to disappear. One day—it's like a miracle—it will disappear." On March 9, as the number of confirmed U.S. COVID-19 cases surpassed 500 and several cities and states prepared to issue stay-at-home orders, the president resisted these measures and insisted that the American people had nothing to worry about. "So last year 37,000 Americans died from the common Flu. It averages between 27,000 and 70,000 per year," he tweeted. "Nothing is shut down, life & the economy go on" (Gilson, Thompson, and Jeffery 2020). By May 3, nearly 22,000 people had died from COVID-19 in the New York City area alone. Infectious disease models suggested that the death toll could have been reduced to 4,300 if control measures had been put in place by March 9 (Glanz and Robertson 2020).

In interviews, press conferences, and public appearances, Trump frequently provided misinformation that contradicted medical experts. Despite evidence that the virus was spreading to new parts of the United States, for instance, Trump repeatedly insisted that the number of COVID-19 cases was declining as the initial patients recovered. "We're going down, not up. We're going very substantially down, not up," he said on February 26 (Leonhardt 2020). "Within a couple of days it's going to be down to close to zero, that's a pretty good job we've done," he added (Gilson, Thompson, and Jeffery 2020). Trump also claimed that a vaccine would be available in a matter of months, ignoring the estimated timetable of one to two years offered by infectious disease experts and pharmaceutical manufacturers. "We'll essentially have a flu shot for this in a fairly quick manner," he declared. "[The drug companies are] going to have vaccines I think relatively soon. And they're going to have something that makes you better, and that's going to actually take place we think even sooner" (Gilson, Thompson, and Jeffery 2020).

By the end of February, when WHO reported more than 85,000 confirmed COVID-19 cases in 55 countries (Leonhardt 2020), the U.S. stock market began dropping due to fears of a global pandemic. Around this time, critics contend that Trump began shifting his approach to the public health crisis. Rather than denying the severity of the situation and offering reassurances, he increasingly moved toward praising his administration's response and blaming his enemies for problems that arose. He claimed that Obama-era regulations delayed the production of testing supplies, for instance, and asserted that Democrats' lax immigration policies allowed the "foreign virus" to enter the United States. "Now the Democrats are politicizing the coronavirus," Trump told supporters at a February 28 rally. "You know that, right? Coronavirus. They're politicizing it. . . . And this is their new hoax." Trump also attacked the mainstream media, claiming that it exaggerated the threat posed by the virus in an attempt to damage his prospects for reelection. "We have a perfectly coordinated and fine tuned plan at the White House for our attack on CoronaVirus," he tweeted on March 8. "The Fake News Media is doing everything possible to make us look bad. Sad!" (Gilson, Thompson, and Jeffery 2020).

In early March, public health experts called for aggressive measures to contain the spread of SARS-CoV-2, such as closing schools and businesses, encouraging people to avoid large gatherings and unnecessary travel, and urging vulnerable populations to wear face masks and adopt social distancing precautions. They noted that the president had a unique platform to publicize and generate support for such measures. Instead, according to critics, Trump often undermined public health guidelines and recommended practices by expressing doubts about their effectiveness or complaining about their impact on the economy. "The inconsistent and sometimes outright incorrect information coming from the White House has left Americans unsure of what, if anything, to do," wrote Leonhardt (2020). Rather than relying on the advice of medical experts, Trump often dismissed it and exaggerated his own scientific knowledge. "I like this stuff. I really get it," he told reporters following a March 6 tour of the CDC. "People are surprised that I understand it. Every one of these doctors said, 'How do you know so much about this?' Maybe I have a natural ability. Maybe I should have done that instead of running for president" (Leonhardt 2020).

By March 10, WHO reported nearly 114,000 coronavirus cases in more than 100 countries. The number of confirmed cases in the United States surpassed 750 that day, as several cities experienced significant outbreaks. Some critics blamed the Trump administration's lack of preparedness and slow response for allowing COVID-19 to spread across the country. "Those two months have meant the difference between many tens of thousands of Americans dying who might otherwise not have died," Rice stated. "[Trump] has demonstrated utter lack of leadership, utter incompetence. And he's been profoundly dishonest about the nature of the threat to the American people by downplaying it, by dismissing it, by comparing it to the flu" (Capehart 2020). Some analysts held the president personally responsible for the shortcomings in his administration's approach to the pandemic. "Trump's utterances between January and the first part of March—denying, minimizing, and peddling junk science as the unfolding disaster cast its shadow—are now legendary," wrote Ghitis. "He acted as if the coronavirus was a political and PR problem that could be fixed with empty reassurances and propaganda, rather than a public health crisis demanding smart and forceful action" (Ghitis 2020).

Further Reading

Blake, Aaron. 2020. "Two Months in the Dark: The Increasingly Damning Timeline of Trump's Coronavirus Response." *Washington Post,* April 21, 2020. https://www.washingtonpost.com/politics/2020/04/07/timeline-trumps -coronavirus-response-is-increasingly-damning/.

Borio, Luciana, and Scott Gottlieb. 2020. "Act Now to Prevent an American Epidemic." *Wall Street Journal,* January 28, 2020. https://www.wsj.com /articles/act-now-to-prevent-an-american-epidemic-11580255335.

Capehart, Jonathan. 2020. "Susan Rice on Trump's Coronavirus Response: 'He Has Cost Thousands of American Lives.'" *Washington Post,* April 6, 2020. https://www.washingtonpost.com/opinions/2020/04/06/susan-rice -trumps-coronavirus-response-he-has-cost-tens-thousands-american -lives/.

CDC. 2020. "First Travel-Related Case of 2019 Novel Coronavirus Detected in United States." Press Release, January 21, 2020. https://www.cdc.gov /media/releases/2020/p0121-novel-coronavirus-travel-case.html.

Eder, Steve, Henry Fountain, Michael H. Keller, Muyi Xiao, and Alexandra Stevenson. 2020. "430,000 People Have Traveled from China to U.S. since Coronavirus Surfaced." *New York Times,* April 4, 2020. https://www .nytimes.com/2020/04/04/us/coronavirus-china-travel-restrictions.html.

Ghitis, Frida. 2020. "Trump Is Fighting a Public Health Crisis with Denial and Self-Promotion." CNN, May 1, 2020. https://www.cnn.com/2020/05/01 /opinions/trump-coronavirus-denial-and-self-promotion-ghitis/index .html.

Gilson, Dave, Laura Thompson, and Clara Jeffery. 2020. "Trump's 100 Days of Deadly Coronavirus Denial." *Mother Jones,* April 29, 2020. https://www .motherjones.com/politics/2020/04/trump-coronavirus-timeline/.

Glanz, James, and Campbell Robertson. 2020. "Lockdown Delays Cost at Least 36,000 Lives, Data Show." *New York Times,* May 20, 2020. https://www .nytimes.com/2020/05/20/us/coronavirus-distancing-deaths.html.

Leonhardt, David. 2020. "A Complete List of Trump's Attempts to Play Down Coronavirus." *New York Times,* March 15, 2020. https://www.nytimes .com/2020/03/15/opinion/trump-coronavirus.html.

Rieder, Rem. 2020. "Contrary to Trump's Claim, a Pandemic Was Widely Expected at Some Point." FactCheck.org, March 20, 2020. https://www .factcheck.org/2020/03/contrary-to-trumps-claim-a-pandemic-was -widely-expected-at-some-point/.

Trump, Donald. 2020. "Remarks by President Trump after Tour of the Centers for Disease Control and Prevention, Atlanta, Georgia." The White House, March 7, 2020. https://www.whitehouse.gov/briefings-statements/remarks -president-trump-tour-centers-disease-control-prevention-atlanta-ga/.

Weber, Peter. 2020. "Trump Wants Praise for His Coronavirus Response. Here It Is." *The Week,* April 25, 2020. https://theweek.com/articles/909198/trump -wants-praise-coronavirus-response-here.

WHO Declares a Global Pandemic (March 11, 2020)

On March 11, 2020, the World Health Organization (WHO) officially designated the COVID-19 outbreak as a global pandemic. By that time, the agency had recorded more than 120,000 cases and 4,300 deaths in 110 countries worldwide. The novel coronavirus SARS-CoV-2 first emerged in

Wuhan, China, in December 2019, and the following month WHO officials declared it a Public Health Emergency of International Concern. The
pandemic designation reflected the continued spread of the disease beyond
a specific community, country, or region.

Some critics charged that the agency waited too long to apply the term
to COVID-19. They claimed that WHO's hesitation allowed world leaders
to remain complacent and avoid taking the aggressive action required to
prevent a pandemic. WHO officials argued that regardless of the termi-
nology used, they had continually stressed the urgent need for a coordinated international response to the virus. "Pandemic is not a word to use
lightly or carelessly. It is a word that, if misused, can cause unreasonable
fear, or unjustified acceptance that the fight is over, leading to unnecessary suffering and death," explained WHO Director General Tedros Adhanom Ghebreyesus. "Describing the situation as a pandemic does not
change WHO's assessment of the threat posed by this coronavirus. It
doesn't change what WHO is doing, and it doesn't change what countries
should do" (Ghebreyesus 2020).

WHO Issues a Wake-Up Call

The announcement on March 11 marked the first time in over a decade
that WHO had declared an infectious disease pandemic, since the H1N1
influenza outbreak of 2009. The agency had resisted applying the term to
several recent outbreaks of Ebola virus, as well as to the previous widespread outbreaks caused by coronaviruses—Severe Acute Respiratory
Syndrome (SARS) and Middle East Respiratory Syndrome (MERS). Some
observers pointed out that WHO's decision to designate swine flu as a
pandemic had come under intense criticism. When the H1N1 virus turned
out to have a very low mortality rate, many governments resented being
asked to devote millions of dollars to purchasing vaccines and implementing containment measures.

In the wake of that experience, WHO leaders revamped the six-phase
pandemic alert process the agency had previously used to describe the
risk level associated with emerging diseases. The steps formerly included
identification of an animal virus with the potential to infect humans
(phase 1), emergence of a human infection caused by an animal virus
(phase 2), reports of scattered cases of disease among humans (phase 3),
evidence of person-to-person transmission and community spread (phase 4),
indications of disease spread beyond a single country (phase 5), and con-
firmation of disease spread beyond a single geographic region (phase 6).
"Each time they went up a stage, it raised alarm. When they finally reached

pandemic stage it caused enormous panic," said Lawrence Gostin, a global health law professor at Georgetown University. "It was so dysfunctional and caused so much fear and panic that WHO abandoned that approach" (Wan 2020).

Rather than moving through distinct phases corresponding to specific criteria in the progression of a disease, WHO officials used a less rigid, less transparent approach to decide when to call COVID-19 a pandemic. According to Michael Ryan, WHO director for health emergencies, there was "no mathematical formula, no algorithm" applied to make the determination (Wan 2020). Instead, WHO officials carefully considered the extent to which the disease had spread as well as its ease of transmission. "I think one of the things people misunderstand when it comes to pandemics is it's not about how severe it is or how many cases there are or even how worried we need to be," said epidemiologist Caitlin Rivers of the Johns Hopkins Center for Health Security. "It's about literal geography" (Wan 2020).

Still, WHO officials understood that the term held serious implications for world leaders and had the potential to generate major political and economic repercussions. The pandemic declaration provided a clear signal that leading experts within the United Nations' health agency anticipated the sustained global spread of COVID-19. "This is a reality check for every government on the planet: Wake up. Get ready," Ryan said. "This virus may be on its way and you need to be ready. You have a duty to your citizens, you have a duty to the world to be ready" (Kopecki et al. 2020).

In his announcement, Ghebreyesus admonished countries for delays in responding to the crisis and warned them to take immediate steps to prepare. "We are deeply concerned both by the alarming levels of spread and severity, and by the alarming levels of inaction," he stated. "We cannot say this loudly enough, or clearly enough, or often enough: all countries can still change the course of this pandemic. . . . Some countries are struggling with a lack of capacity. Some countries are struggling with a lack of resources. Some countries are struggling with a lack of resolve" (Ghebreyesus 2020).

Ghebreyesus urged world leaders to put emergency response systems in place, including travel restrictions, quarantines, and testing and contact tracing protocols. He also recommended training hospital workers in safe treatment methods and informing citizens about the best ways to protect themselves. Finally, the director general warned countries to anticipate economic and social disruptions due to the pandemic and to take steps to secure human rights. "This is not just a public health crisis, it is a crisis that will touch every sector," he declared. "If countries detect, test, treat, isolate, trace, and mobilize their people in the response, those with a handful of cases can prevent those cases becoming clusters, and those clusters becoming community transmission" (Ghebreyesus 2020).

Ghebreyesus ended on a note of encouragement and optimism, pointing out that calling COVID-19 a pandemic did not imply that the world had lost its fight against the disease. "There's been so much attention on one word," he said. "Let me give you some other words that matter much more, and that are much more actionable. Prevention. Preparedness. Public health. Political leadership. And most of all, people. We're in this together, to do the right things with calm and protect the citizens of the world. It's doable" (Ghebreyesus 2020).

Contrasting Strategies to Stop the Spread

By the time WHO declared COVID-19 a pandemic, confirmed cases had appeared on every continent except Antarctica. Even as China made significant progress toward containing the initial outbreak, the number of infections outside of China grew by a factor of 13 within a two-week period. New hot spots emerged in Italy, with more than 10,000 cases and 630 deaths, as well as in Iran, with 9,000 cases, and South Korea, with nearly 8,000 cases. The coronavirus also showed signs of spreading within the United States, which recorded more than 1,000 cases in 36 states. On the plus side, according to WHO data, those five countries accounted for 90 percent of all cases worldwide at the time of the pandemic declaration, and more than 80 countries still had no confirmed cases (Kopecki et al. 2020).

Public health experts contrasted the national responses to the coronavirus pandemic in Italy and South Korea. Italy's reactive approach allowed COVID-19 to develop into the country's biggest crisis since World War II, with 237,000 cases and 34,400 deaths by mid-June in a total population of 60 million. South Korea, on the other hand, adopted a proactive approach that effectively contained the disease within a month, so it recorded only 12,000 cases and fewer than 300 deaths by mid-June in a total population of 51 million.

SARS-CoV-2 swept across Italy in a matter of weeks, overwhelming its health care system and forcing doctors to ration life-saving equipment and care among the patients they deemed most likely to survive. Following the first confirmed case on February 21, Italian leaders did not recognize the threat quickly enough and downplayed the severity of the virus in public statements and actions. In a display intended to calm fears, for instance, several high-profile Italian politicians organized a public handshaking in

Milan. One of the participants tested positive for COVID-19 a week later. Italian leaders initially resisted taking aggressive action to stop the spread of the coronavirus. "The most effective time to take strong action is extremely early, when the threat appears to be small—or even before there are any cases," noted a panel of experts in the *Harvard Business Review*. "But if the intervention actually works, it will appear in retrospect as if the strong actions were an overreaction. This is a game many politicians don't want to play" (Pisano, Sadun, and Zanini 2020).

Rather than organizing a nationwide, systematic response, the Italian government issued a series of decrees that gradually increased social restrictions and expanded lockdown areas until these measures finally applied to the entire country. As a result, the lockdown measures followed, rather than prevented, the spread of the virus—especially when thousands of citizens responded to regional restrictions by rushing to unaffected regions. Although some areas of Italy, such as Veneto, experienced success in containing the virus through proactive test-and-trace protocols, the central government failed to learn from and apply these strategies nationally. "An effective response to the virus needs to be orchestrated as a coherent system of actions taken simultaneously," the *Harvard Business Review* panel explained. "Testing is effective when it's combined with rigorous contact tracing, and tracing is effective as long as it is combined with an effective communication system that collects and disseminates information on the movements of potentially infected people, and so forth" (Pisano, Sadun, and Zanini 2020).

South Korea's response to COVID-19 demonstrated the effectiveness of these strategies, which its government and people had learned by dealing with previous outbreaks of SARS in 2002, H1N1 influenza in 2009, and MERS in 2015. The MERS experience prompted South Korean leaders to institute a new infectious disease prevention protocol that featured early testing, extensive contact tracing using cell phone location data and closed-circuit television footage, community health measures to isolate new patients, and open communication to build public trust and ensure full cooperation with containment policies.

In conjunction with this pandemic preparedness system, South Korea began developing and mass producing diagnostic test kits immediately after its first confirmed case appeared in late January. Public health officials established 600 drive-through testing stations that provided results in 10 minutes, and by early March they had tested 145,000 people. South Korea also instituted a high-tech contact-tracing system to warn local residents when they may have been exposed to COVID-19. "They'll send out an alert saying that there were X number of new confirmed cases today, if any, and that you can check their routes on the district website," said Seoul resident Yung In Chae. "On the website, each patient is identified [by] their gender and their age. They also note, with asterisks, whether their houses have been disinfected, whether there were contacts, and whether they were wearing masks the entire time" (Thompson 2020). Public health officials used this data to identify and isolate potential contacts to prevent the spread of the virus. South Korea also enacted a community health approach that treated elderly and seriously ill patients in hospitals, sent moderately ill people to isolation facilities for medical monitoring, and kept asymptomatic patients in self-quarantine at home.

Public health officials held daily briefings to keep people informed about the latest developments and encourage them to adopt such measures as wearing face masks and social distancing. Voluntary compliance with these measures enabled South Korea to avoid closing businesses and issuing strict stay-at-home orders. "We were never on lockdown," said Seoul resident Paul Choi. "But citizens have taken it upon ourselves to stay inside. We're very careful to wash our hands and keep our distance. Almost everybody is wearing masks. If you don't wear masks, you get looks on the street" (Thompson 2020). South Korea's coordinated response to the crisis stopped the spread of COVID-19 within a month. Between the end of February—when South Korea had the largest number of confirmed cases outside of China—and the end of March, the number of new daily cases fell by 90 percent. At the time WHO declared COVID-19 a global pandemic, South Korea and the United States had both recorded around 90 deaths due to the disease. While South Korea lost a total of 85 more people during the month of April, however, the United States averaged that many COVID-19 deaths per hour, for a total of 62,000 that month (Thompson 2020).

Further Reading

Chappell, Bill. 2020. "Coronavirus: COVID-19 Is Now Officially a Pandemic, WHO Says." NPR, March 11, 2020. https://www.npr.org/sections/goats andsoda/2020/03/11/814474930/coronavirus-covid-19-is-now-officially -a-pandemic-who-says.

Ducharme, Jamie. 2020. "World Health Organization Declares COVID-19 a 'Pandemic.' Here's What That Means." *Time,* March 11, 2020. https://time .com/5791661/who-coronavirus-pandemic-declaration/.

Ghebreyesus, Tedros Adhanom. 2020. "WHO Director-General's Opening Remarks at the Media Briefing on COVID-19." World Health Organization, March 11, 2020. https://www.who.int/dg/speeches/detail/who-director -general-s-opening-remarks-at-the-media-briefing-on-covid-19—11 -march-2020.

Kopecki, Dawn, Berkeley Lovelace Jr., William Feuer, and Noah Higgins-Dunn. 2020. "World Health Organization Declares the Coronavirus a Global Pandemic." CNBC, March 11, 2020. https://www.cnbc.com/2020/03/11 /who-declares-the-coronavirus-outbreak-a-global-pandemic.html.

Pisano, Gary P., Raffaella Sadun, and Michele Zanini. 2020. "Lessons from Italy's Response to Coronavirus." *Harvard Business Review,* March 27, 2020. https://hbr.org/2020/03/lessons-from-italys-response-to-coronavirus.

Thompson, Derek. 2020. "What's Behind South Korea's COVID-19 Exceptionalism?" *Atlantic,* May 6, 2020. https://www.theatlantic.com/ideas/archive /2020/05/whats-south-koreas-secret/611215/.

Wan, William. 2020. "WHO Declares a Pandemic of Coronavirus Disease COVID-19." *Washington Post,* March 11, 2020. https://www.washington post.com/health/2020/03/11/who-declares-pandemic-coronavirus -disease-covid-19.

American Sports Leagues Suspend Play (March 11–12, 2020)

On March 11, 2020—the same day that the World Health Organization (WHO) classified COVID-19 as a global pandemic—a pivotal event occurred that forced millions of formerly complacent Americans to confront the fact that the rapidly spreading virus would have a broad and lasting impact on their daily lives. The National Basketball Association (NBA) announced plans to suspend play immediately and cancel the remainder of the season because an unnamed player had tested positive for SARS-CoV-2. "The NBA will use this hiatus to determine next steps for moving forward in regard to the coronavirus pandemic," the league commissioner said in a statement (Hanna, Almasy, and Close 2020). The next day, most other professional and collegiate sports leagues followed the NBA's lead and halted their seasons. The sudden and unexpected stoppage of virtually all organized sporting events made fans understand the gravity of the public health crisis facing the nation in a way that political leaders, medical experts, and news reports had failed to convey.

Sports Adjust to the Pandemic

Before the NBA shut down, American sports leagues had offered little indication that they planned to make significant changes to their operations in response to the COVID-19 pandemic. As public health experts began recommending that people observe such commonsense precautions as washing hands frequently, bumping elbows rather than shaking hands, and avoiding large gatherings, some organizing bodies discussed how to translate these ideas into actions to keep sports fans and athletes safe. Early speculation centered on the idea of continuing to hold sporting events but either limiting the number of spectators or banning spectators entirely to prevent close contact between people in crowds.

The first U.S. sporting event to be played without fans due to COVID-19 took place on March 6 in Amherst, Massachusetts. It was a Division III women's college basketball game between Rowan University and the U.S. Merchant Marine Academy. "It was an empty arena, no energy. You had to pull it from yourself," Rowan Coach Demetrius Poles recalled. "We didn't get anything. It was just whistles and sneakers" (Sheinin 2020). As the National Collegiate Athletic Association (NCAA) prepared for its annual March Madness men's basketball championship tournament to begin the following week, officials developed contingency plans in case they had to hold contests without anyone in attendance. Major professional sporting events went on as scheduled, however, and some high-profile athletes rejected the notion of playing in empty arenas. "I play for the fans; that's what it's all about," said Los Angeles Lakers star LeBron James. "If I show up to the arena and there ain't no fans there, I ain't playing" (Sheinin 2020).

Two days later, coronavirus concerns prompted the cancellation of a major U.S. sporting event for the first time. As the number of confirmed cases in the United States surpassed 550, officials called off the BNP Paribas Open tennis tournament in Indian Wells, California. Although the athletes probably could have competed safely on opposite ends of the court, organizers wanted to avoid the large crowds the event typically attracted. Some players had already arrived at the venue and expressed dismay that the tournament was canceled without their input. "We were just told very abruptly that the tournament was canceled," said Canadian player Vasek Pospisil. "It's kind of a weird situation because you also understand the gravity of the coronavirus and you need to respect that. At the same time, I think it's just a confusing time for everybody. Emotionally, it's tough to really pinpoint how we're feeling because it's out of our control" (Sheinin 2020).

On March 9, as the number of confirmed COVID-19 deaths in the United States reached 26, American professional sports leagues took steps to keep athletes separate from fans and members of the media. Major League Baseball (MLB), Major League Soccer (MLS), the NBA, and the National Hockey League (NHL) issued a joint statement announcing the immediate closure of team locker rooms and clubhouses to nonessential personnel. To minimize close contact with the public, only players and team employees were allowed to enter these spaces, while media access shifted to designated interview rooms where members of the press were asked to maintain an appropriate social distance of 6 feet from players and coaches. Some teams also provided extra hand sanitizer dispensers, performed additional cleaning and disinfection of public areas, and urged athletes to avoid high-fives, handshakes, and autograph sessions with fans.

On March 10, as the number of confirmed COVID-19 cases in the United States surpassed 1,000, the Ivy League Conference announced its decision to cancel its men's and women's basketball tournaments. Many athletes and coaches expressed disappointment, frustration, or disgust with the decision. "I just think it's an overreaction, from what we know now," said University of Pennsylvania coach Steve Donahue, who worried about the impact on student-athletes in their final year of NCAA eligibility. "All the things they've worked for since they were 7, 8 years old—to get it torn away like this seems really unfair" (Sheinin 2020). Harvard University player Bryce Aiken asserted that teams understood the health risks and should have been given the option to play. "Horrible, horrible, horrible decision and total disregard for the players and teams that have put their hearts into this season," he tweeted (Sheinin 2020).

The situation evolved rapidly on March 11. The Big Ten Conference held the first two games of its men's basketball tournament in Indianapolis with spectators in attendance. During the second game of the day between the Indiana Hoosiers and Nebraska Cornhuskers, however, Nebraska Coach Fred Hoiberg appeared visibly ill on the bench. Fans and television announcers watched anxiously as players and coaches seated nearby applied hand sanitizer. After the game, the Nebraska team stayed isolated in the locker room while Hoiberg went to the hospital, where he was diagnosed with influenza A rather than COVID-19. The close call spurred the Big Ten to announce that all remaining games of the conference tournament would be played without fans in attendance. Most other college conferences immediately followed suit, and the NCAA quickly announced that the March Madness championship tournament would exclude spectators as well. The Ivy League went a step further and announced the cancellation of all spring sports.

The NBA Makes a Stunning Announcement

Four of the six NBA games scheduled to be played on March 11 tipped off as usual with fans in attendance. The other two games—featuring the Utah Jazz at the Oklahoma Thunder, and the New Orleans Pelicans at the Sacramento Kings—halted abruptly as the teams completed their pregame warmups. At Chesapeake Energy Arena in Oklahoma City, officials herded the players off the court and into their locker rooms while a public address announcer told spectators to go home. "Due to unforeseen circumstances the game has been postponed," the announcer stated. "Good night, fans" (Hanna, Almasy, and Close 2020). Less than an hour later, the NBA commissioner issued a statement saying that the league would suspend play immediately and cancel the rest of the season because an unnamed player had tested positive for SARS-CoV-2.

It soon became clear that the player in question was Rudy Gobert, an all-star center for the Utah Jazz. A viral video quickly emerged from a news conference Gobert attended two days earlier, after the NBA had imposed restrictions on media access to locker rooms, in which he answered questions about how players were coping with coronavirus concerns. "There's not much we can do right now," he replied. "We're not going to stop touching—stop saying hi to each other or stop giving each other high-fives. But just being aware of it. And try to have some hygiene—a little more hygiene, especially with the hands" (Sheinin 2020). As the interviews concluded, Gobert stood up, grinned at reporters, and proceeded to touch all of the microphones, cell phones, and tape recorders arrayed on the table in front of him before leaving the room. Although Gobert intended it as a lighthearted gesture in defiance of what he viewed as ridiculous precautions, video footage of the stunt generated widespread outrage following his diagnosis. Critics pointed out that he could infect other people even if he never developed symptoms, and that the coronavirus could live on surfaces he touched for hours or days.

Gobert apologized for his actions on social media. "At the time, I had no idea I was even infected," he wrote. "I was careless and make no excuse. I hope my story serves as a warning and causes everyone to take this seriously. I will do whatever I can to support using my experience as way to educate others and prevent the spread of this virus" (Lupica 2020). One of Gobert's teammates, guard Donovan Mitchell, also tested positive for COVID-19. The NBA asked the other Jazz players and coaches, as well as members of the four teams that had faced the Jazz in the preceding week—the Boston Celtics, Detroit Pistons, Toronto Raptors, and Washington Wizards—to self-quarantine for 14 days as a precautionary measure.

A survey of 1,000 sports fans conducted by the online ticket retailer TickPick found that the cancellation of the NBA season—along with the media coverage of Gobert's diagnosis—helped raise awareness of the threat posed by the coronavirus pandemic. Fully 84 percent of respondents said these events made them take COVID-19 more seriously, while two-thirds said they felt more anxious about the spread of the disease afterward (Reimer 2020). Some sportswriters described Gobert as an "accidental hero" and claimed that he saved lives by demonstrating how easily SARS-CoV-2 could be transmitted. "He was us. He wasn't concerned about coronavirus, neither getting it nor spreading it. He was cavalier about the possibilities, even to the point of touching teammates and their belongings prior to his diagnosis," wrote Jenni Carlson of the *Oklahoman*. "He was the change agent for how Americans think about coronavirus. Millions of us came to better understand its impact and its reach, and the result has been unprecedented actions to try and get it under control. Because of that, fewer people will be infected, and because of that, more people will be able to get treatment and survive" (Carlson 2020).

The shocking events in the world of basketball continued on March 12, as one college conference after another abruptly canceled their championship tournaments—in some cases with teams already on the court in empty arenas. Officials stopped a Big East men's quarterfinal game at halftime, for instance, with St. John's leading Creighton by a score of 38-35. Both the Big Ten and Atlantic Ten Conferences called off tournament games while teams were performing pre-game warmups. The defending NCAA Division I national champion women's basketball team from Baylor University learned that their season had ended prematurely while waiting on the tarmac to take off for the Big Twelve tournament in Kansas City. Later that day, the NCAA officially canceled both the men's and women's March Madness tournaments, as well all spring collegiate sports seasons.

Other Sports Cancel or Postpone Seasons

Following the announcements by the NBA and NCAA, every other major American sport quickly fell in line and suspended, canceled, or postponed individual events or entire seasons in response to the coronavirus pandemic. MLB canceled all remaining spring training games and delayed Opening Day of the 2020 season by at least two weeks. "It's got to happen," said Los Angeles Dodgers pitcher David Price. "This is so much bigger than sports. I've got two kids" (Sheinin 2020). The NHL suspended the remainder of its season and canceled the upcoming playoffs. "Following last night's news that an NBA player has tested positive for coronavirus—and given that our leagues share so many facilities and locker rooms and it now seems likely that some member of the NHL community would test positive at some point—it is no longer appropriate to try to continue to play games at this time," said NHL Commissioner Gary Bettman (Andone 2020).

Major League Soccer announced a 30-day suspension of its season. The Professional Golfers Association (PGA) Tour canceled the Players Championship and all other events through April 5, and Augusta National

Golf Course officials postponed the Masters, which had been scheduled to begin on April 9. "Ultimately, the health and well-being of everyone associated with these events and the citizens of the Augusta community led us to this decision," Augusta Chairman Fred Ridley explained (Andone 2020). NASCAR announced that it would hold upcoming races without fans in attendance. Organizers of the Boston Marathon, which had been scheduled to take place on April 20, decided to postpone the event until September 14. "Our expectation and the hope right now is that this date will get us to a safer place in relation to the spread of the coronavirus," said Boston Mayor Marty Walsh (Andone 2020).

The last major sporting event to alter its schedule in response to the COVID-19 pandemic was the 2020 Olympic Games, scheduled to begin in mid-July in Tokyo, Japan. Organizers noted that the Games had only been canceled three times previously—in 1916, 1940, and 1944—due to world wars. Before the end of March, however, Japanese Prime Minister Shinzo Abe and International Olympic Committee President Thomas Bach announced plans to postpone the Tokyo 2020 Olympics until 2021. Although the postponement was estimated to cost organizers up to $25 billion, they noted that the pandemic made a mass gathering of athletes and fans from different countries extremely dangerous. Organizers expressed hope that the 2021 Olympics could help the world recover from the impact of the coronavirus. "The Olympic Games in Tokyo could stand as a beacon of hope to the world during these troubled times," the IOC statement noted, "[and] the Olympic flame could become the light at the end of the tunnel in which the world finds itself at present" (Cohen 2020).

Observers noted that the wholesale cancellation of sporting events marked an unprecedented moment in U.S. history. "At some of America's worst times, sports has been there to restore a sense of normalcy. That was President Franklin D. Roosevelt's argument for pushing baseball to play on during World War II and the NFL's and MLB's reason to return after short hiatuses in the aftermath of the 9/11 attacks," Dave Sheinin wrote in the *Washington Post*. "But this time is different because of the spread of an invisible virus. COVID-19 changed everything. Playing through this crisis would not have been a solution; it would have been a major part of the problem" (Sheinin 2020). American sports fans got by in the absence of sports by watching reruns of classic games, dissecting their home teams' draft selections, perusing their favorite athletes' social media posts and podcasts, or following obscure sports that could be contested with social-distancing protocols in place, such as ax throwing, cornhole, cup stacking, and miniature golf.

Further Reading

Andone, Dakin. 2020. "Major Sports Leagues in the U.S. Halt Play or Exclude Fans over Coronavirus Outbreaks." CNN, March 13, 2020. https://www .cnn.com/2020/03/12/us/us-sports-coronavirus-response/index.html.

Carlson, Jenni. 2020. "Coronavirus in Oklahoma: Yes, Jazz Star Rudy Gobert Was a Goob, but He's also Become an Accidental Hero." *Oklahoman,* March 15, 2020. https://oklahoman.com/article/5657635/coronavirus-in -oklahoma-yes-jazz-star-rudy-gobert-was-a-goob-but-hes-also-become -an-accidental-hero.

Cohen, Kelly. 2020. "Tokyo 2020 Olympics Officially Postponed until 2021." ESPN, March 24, 2020. https://www.espn.com/olympics/story/_/id/2894 6033/tokyo-olympics-officially-postponed-2021.

Hanna, Jason, Steve Almasy, and David Close. 2020. "Utah Jazz Center Rudy Gobert, Found to Have Coronavirus, Apologizes for Possibly Endanger- ing People." CNN, March 12, 2020. https://www.cnn.com/2020/03/12 /us/nba-season-suspended-utah-jazz-coronavirus-spt-trnd/index.html.

Lupica, Mike. 2020. "Rudy Gobert Saved the World." *New York Daily News,* March 13, 2020. https://www.nydailynews.com/sports/basketball/ny-rudy -gobert-coronavirus-nba-shutdown-20200313-parqbv2y5vehrp2csqqrkr sydu-story.html.

Reimer, Alex. 2020. "Coronavirus Reactions: Sports Fans Took Virus Much More Seriously after Leagues Canceled, Survey Says." *Forbes,* April 9, 2020. https://www.forbes.com/sites/alexreimer/2020/04/09/sports-fans-took -coronavirus-much-more-seriously-after-leagues-canceled-survey-says /#7b1a2a041ffc.

Sheinin, Dave. 2020. "The Week the Coronavirus Ground the Sports World to a Halt." *Washington Post,* March 14, 2020. https://www.washingtonpost .com/sports/2020/03/14/sports-cancellations-timeline-coronavirus/?arc 404=true.

Vera, Amir. 2020. "Pro Sports Leagues Like the NBA and MLB Will Restrict Locker Room Access Indefinitely to Combat Coronavirus." CNN, March 9, 2020. https://www.cnn.com/2020/03/09/us/sports-leagues-no-locker-room -access-spt/index.html.

Stock Market Crash Reflects Coronavirus Concerns (March 16, 2020)

As COVID-19 cases began appearing around the world in the first quarter of 2020, the growing public health crisis created unprecedented challenges for national economies. To prevent the spread of the virus, businesses and industries shut down, workers lost jobs, consumers stayed home and curtailed purchasing, and governments experienced budget shortfalls as their tax bases declined and the costs of responding to the emergency rose. Leading economic experts acknowledged that the global pandemic put them in uncharted territory and made it difficult to predict the severity and duration of its impact.

Stock markets around the world reflected public fears and uncertainty by showing extreme volatility in the early months of 2020. In the United States, for instance, the Dow Jones Industrial Average reached record highs in February before losing one-third of its value in March through a series of crashes—including the largest one-day point drop in history on March 16. Although the Dow largely recovered in April and May, it dropped once again in June as hopes for a quick economic recovery sank in the face of a second wave of coronavirus outbreaks. Some critics charged that economic concerns drove U.S. political leaders to lift containment measures too soon, which allowed a resurgence of COVID-19 cases.

Unprecedented Stock Market Volatility

After a decade of growth, the world economy showed some signs of slowing down in 2019, including declining manufacturing output, increasing corporate debt, and rising geopolitical tensions over trade policy. Yet the three main U.S. stock market indicators—the Dow Jones Industrial Average, the NASDAQ Composite Index, and the S&P 500 Index—remained strong through 2019 and into early 2020. In fact, all three indices set record highs at the end of trading on February 12, 2020. In public statements and social media posts, President Donald Trump often equated high stock market values with the overall health of the U.S. economy and attributed both to his administration's successful fiscal policies. According to *New York Times* opinion writer Neil Irwin, Trump "spent the last three years personalizing much of what happens in the markets and the economy, saying that the soaring stock values under his watch are a reflection of his special ability, and a central part of his case for re-election in November" (Irwin 2020).

By the end of February, the World Health Organization (WHO) reported more than 85,000 confirmed COVID-19 cases in 55 countries (Leonhardt 2020). As the novel coronavirus spread, global stock market values began falling as investors grew worried about the potential for a pandemic to disrupt the world economy. Trump and other administration officials downplayed the severity of the public health crisis and promised to minimize its economic impact in an effort to reassure nervous investors. "The Coronavirus is very much under control in the USA," the president tweeted on February 26. "We are in contact with everyone and all relevant countries. CDC & World Health have been working hard and very smart. Stock Market starting to look very good to me!" (Irwin 2020).

Trump's optimistic outlook failed to arrest the downward momentum of the U.S. and world stock markets, which on February 28 reported their largest weekly declines since the 2008 global financial crisis and recession. The president claimed that U.S. public health officials counteracted his positive message with alarmist statements about COVID-19 spreading within the United States. "It's not so much of a question of if this will happen anymore, but rather more of a question of exactly when this will happen," said Dr. Nancy Messonnier, director of the National Center for Immunization and Respiratory Diseases, at a February 25 press briefing. "We are asking the American public to prepare for the expectation that this could be bad" (Irwin 2020). Trump also claimed that the media exaggerated the impact of the coronavirus in an attempt to harm his reelection chances. On February 26, he asserted on Twitter that mainstream news outlets were "doing everything possible to make the Coronavirus look as bad as possible, including panicking markets. . . . USA in great shape!" (Irwin 2020).

Trump and other administration officials insisted that the volatility in the stock market reflected a short-term correction rather than a long-term response to coronavirus concerns. "I think the stock market is something I know a lot about," the president stated in a news conference. "I think the stock market will recover. The economy is very strong" (Irwin 2020). White House economic adviser Larry Kudlow described the market downturn as temporary and argued that it offered a great opportunity for investors. "The virus story is not going to last forever," he said. "To me, if you are an investor out there and you have a long-term point of view, I would suggest very seriously taking a look at the market, the stock market, that is a lot cheaper than it was a week or two ago" (Irwin 2020).

The economic news got worse in early March, as COVID-19 outbreaks triggered economic crises in country after country around the world. The enactment of travel restrictions and stay-at-home orders to contain the spread of the virus disrupted supply chains and labor markets and contributed to business closures and rising unemployment rates. In addition, plummeting global demand for petroleum sparked an oil price war between Russia and Saudi Arabia that further destabilized commodities markets worldwide. On March 9, which became known as Black Monday, these factors combined to trigger a dramatic one-day decline in the value of world stock markets. On Wall Street, the S&P 500 fell so rapidly—losing 7 percent of its value within the first four minutes of trading—that it activated a regulatory tool known as a "circuit breaker" to temporarily halt trading. By the end of the day, the Dow had set a new single-day record by dropping 2,013 points.

On March 11—the day that WHO declared COVID-19 a global pandemic—Trump made a nationally televised speech from the Oval

Office for only the second time in his presidency. Citing the rapid spread of the coronavirus, he announced a 30-day suspension of travel to the United States from countries in Europe, with the exception of the United Kingdom. "Taking early intense action, we have seen dramatically fewer cases of the virus in the United States than are now present in Europe," he explained. "The European Union failed to take the same precautions and restrict travel from China and other hot spots. As a result, a large number of new clusters in the United States were seeded by travelers from Europe. After consulting with our top government health professionals, I have decided to take several strong but necessary actions to protect the health and well-being of all Americans" (Trump 2020).

In addition to the travel restrictions, Trump noted that he signed a bill providing $8.3 billion in emergency funding to the Centers for Disease Control and Prevention (CDC) and other agencies to support work on coronavirus vaccines, treatments, and testing. The president also encouraged the American people to help slow the spread of COVID-19 by practicing good hygiene, including washing hands, disinfecting surfaces, covering coughs and sneezes, and staying home when sick. Finally, Trump promised to provide economic relief to help businesses and workers cope with the pandemic. "This is not a financial crisis," he stated. "This is just a temporary moment of time that we will overcome together as a nation and as a world" (Trump 2020).

Critics claimed that Trump's address did little to calm public fears about the COVID-19 pandemic and instead added an element of uncertainty to the federal response. Although Trump initially said the new travel restrictions applied to trade goods originating in Europe, this turned out to be a misstatement. His announcement also created confusion about whether the travel restrictions only applied only to foreign nationals or whether they also affected Americans traveling or living abroad. The lack of clarity prompted thousands of Americans to risk contracting the virus by packing into European airports in a chaotic rush to return to the United States. Critics also noted that Trump alienated some European allies by failing to warn them in advance of his intention to impose travel restrictions.

Trump's speech also failed to reassure stock market analysts and investors. The following day, March 12—which became known as Black Thursday—the Dow fell by a record 2,353 points, losing 10 percent of its value. Wall Street experienced a brief rally on March 13, when Trump declared a national public health emergency. This action, which released $50 billion in preparedness funding and mobilized additional federal resources to combat the coronavirus, spurred a 1,985-point increase in the Dow.

When the U.S. stock market reopened for trading on March 16, however, the Dow dropped by 2,997 points—setting another record for the largest single-day point loss in history. On that day, which became known as Black Monday II, all three Wall Street indices fell by more than 12 percent. The roller-coaster ride continued a week later, when Congress announced progress toward passing a $2 trillion economic stimulus package and Trump expressed determination to "have the country opened up and raring to go by Easter," prompting a 2,117-point surge in the Dow (Barrabi 2020). Overall, however, global stock markets finished the month of March down 25 to 30 percent from their peak values in February.

Pressure to Reopen the U.S. Economy

The U.S. stock market continued to fluctuate in April and May as the spread of COVID-19 across the country triggered a virtual shutdown of the American economy. From its record high value of 29,000 in February, the Dow lost 34 percent of its value in March, then regained 25 percent of its value in April. On May 26, the Dow surpassed 25,000 again on the strength of low interest rates, federal credit guarantees, and promising news in the quest to develop a vaccine to prevent COVID-19. "Since the beginning of the crisis, stock prices seem to be running wild," noted analysts from the Centre for Economic Policy Research. "They first ignored the pandemic, then panicked when Europe became its epicenter. Now, they are behaving as if the millions of people infected, the 400,000 deaths, and the containment of half the world's population will have no economic impact after all" (Capelle-Blancard and Desroziers 2020).

By June, however, states that reopened their economies began experiencing a second wave of coronavirus cases. As hopes for a quick economic recovery faded, the Dow dropped 1,861 points on June 11. Economists noted that the volatility demonstrated by the U.S. stock market in response to the COVID-19 pandemic was unprecedented, surpassing that seen during some of the worst economic crises in history. They also pointed out that investors had not reacted strongly during previous infectious disease outbreaks, such as SARS, Ebola, H1N1, or even the 1918 influenza pandemic. Experts attributed the stock market's significant response to COVID-19 to the severity of the pandemic, the rapid dissemination of information online, the interconnectedness of the global economy, and the harmful economic impact of lockdown measures imposed to prevent the virus from spreading. "The healthcare rationale for travel restrictions, social-distancing mandates, and other containment policies is clear," according to a Northwestern University analysis. "These policies also bring great economic damage. Recent stock-market behavior is an early and visible reflection of the (expected) damage" (Baker et al. 2020).

Since Trump often took credit for high stock market values and positive economic conditions, he also risked taking the blame—and harming his chances for reelection—if his administration's response to the pandemic failed to prevent a stock market crash and a severe recession. According to critics, Trump's concern about the economic impact of lockdown measures drove him to pressure states to lift restrictions and reopen for business before the virus had been contained. "It's understandable that the administration, in an election year, is focused on keeping the stock market and the economy strong," said political consultant Michael Steel. "But they risk creating the impression that they're more focused on the economic impact of the virus than effective public health measures" (Irwin 2020). Even as the number of confirmed COVID-19 cases in the United States neared 2.5 million in June, administration officials rejected the idea of reestablishing containment policies. "We can't shut down the economy again," said Treasury Secretary Steve Mnuchin (Imbert and Li 2020). Critics charged that the nation could not hope to make a full economic recovery until it got the public health crisis fully under control.

Further Reading

Baker, Scott R., Nicholas Bloom, Steven J. Davis, Kyle Kost, Marco Sammon, and Tasaneeya Viratyosin. 2020. "The Unprecedented Stock Market Reaction to COVID-19." *Kellogg Insight,* April 1, 2020. https://insight.kellogg.north western.edu/article/what-explains-the-unprecedented-stock-market -reaction-to-covid-19.

Barrabi, Thomas. 2020. "The Dow's Biggest Single-Day Gains and Losses in History." Fox Business, June 11, 2020. https://www.foxbusiness.com/markets /the-dows-biggest-single-day-drops-in-history.

Capelle-Blancard, Gunther, and Adrien Desroziers. 2020. "The Stock Market and the Economy: Insights from the COVID-19 Crisis." VoxEU, June 19, 2020. https://voxeu.org/article/stock-market-and-economy-insights-covid -19-crisis.

Forsyth, Randall W. 2020. "Trump's Response to Coronavirus Boosted the Stock Market. The U.S. Is Coming Up Short." *Barron's,* March 14, 2020. https:// www.barrons.com/articles/coming-up-short-in-response-to-the-virus -crisis-11584144198.

Imbert, Fred, and Yun Li. 2020. "Stocks Suffer Their Worst Day since March, with the Dow Plunging More Than 1,800 Points." CNBC, June 10, 2020. https://www.cnbc.com/2020/06/10/stock-market-futures-open-to-close -news.html.

Irwin, Neil. 2020. "Coronavirus Shows the Problem with Trump's Stock Market Boasting." *New York Times,* February 26, 2020. https://www.nytimes.com /2020/02/26/upshot/coronavirus-trump-stock-market.html.

Leonhardt, David. 2020. "A Complete List of Trump's Attempts to Play Down Coronavirus." *New York Times,* March 15, 2020. https://www.nytimes .com/2020/03/15/opinion/trump-coronavirus.html.

Trump, Donald. 2020. "Remarks by President Trump in Address to the Nation." The White House, March 11, 2020. https://www.whitehouse.gov/briefings -statements/remarks-president-trump-address-nation/.

Coronavirus Task Force Holds Daily Briefings (March 16–April 24, 2020)

For nearly six weeks, from March 16 through April 24, President Donald Trump participated in daily press briefings held by the White House Coronavirus Task Force. These briefings—carried live on television news channels and online news sites—provided the media and the public with up-to-date information about the COVID-19 pandemic and the federal government's response to it. "Millions and millions of Americans tune in each day to hear directly from President Trump and appreciate his leadership, unprecedented coronavirus response, and confident outlook for America's future," said White House press secretary Kayleigh McEnany (Pesce 2020). Some observers noted that Trump's appearance at the briefings marked a shift in his administration's approach to the coronavirus. After spending February and early March downplaying the severity of the public health crisis, the president acknowledged the urgency of the situation and began promoting measures intended to contain the spread of the virus.

In the eyes of critics, however, Trump's participation in the daily press briefings did little to inform or reassure the public and often amounted to a self-serving form of political theater. Rather than focusing on the COVID-19 pandemic, Trump often used the platform to praise his administration's performance, attack his political opponents, engage in verbal sparring with reporters, and tout signs of a quick economic recovery. Critics charged that the president repeatedly made false or misleading statements about the coronavirus and challenged the advice of medical experts. Some viewers claimed that Trump used the task force briefings as a replacement for his campaign rallies and questioned whether the media should provide free coverage to such partisan events. On April 25— one day after he made controversial comments about injecting disinfectants to treat COVID-19 infections—Trump announced his intention to step away from the briefings.

The White House Coronavirus Task Force

Trump established the White House Coronavirus Task Force on January 29, nine days after the first confirmed case of COVID-19 appeared in the United States. It initially consisted of 12 members, including Department of Health and Human Services Secretary Alex Azar, National Institute of Allergy and Infectious Diseases Director Anthony Fauci, Centers for Disease Control and Prevention Director Robert Redfield, and National Security Adviser Robert O'Brien. Its original mission was to "monitor, contain, and mitigate the spread of the virus, while ensuring that the American people have the most accurate and up-to-date health and travel information" (Santucci 2020).

On February 26, Trump announced that Vice President Mike Pence would serve as chair of the task force, assuming the role formerly held by Azar. "The president wanted to make it clear to the American people that we're going to bring a whole of government approach to this," Pence explained (Santucci 2020). Some observers praised the move, claiming that it reflected the administration's growing prioritization of the COVID-19 crisis. As governor of Indiana, supporters pointed out, Pence dealt with the emergence of the first MERS case in the United States in 2014. Yet critics questioned the vice president's qualifications to coordinate the national response to a public health emergency. In 2015, they noted, Indiana experienced an epidemic of HIV infections among intravenous drug users. Pence initially rejected a needle-exchange program shown by CDC medical experts to reduce infection rates, comparing it to "handing out drug paraphernalia," before eventually bowing to a public backlash and allowing the program to proceed (Santucci 2020).

Upon taking over as chair, Pence expanded the task force to include Deborah Birx, a respected immunologist and AIDS researcher, as the coronavirus response coordinator. He also added several other members to the group in late February and early March, including U.S. Surgeon General Jerome Adams, Secretary of the Treasury Steve Mnuchin, National Economic Council Director Larry Kudrow, Secretary of Housing and Urban Development Ben Carson, FDA Commissioner Stephen Hahn, and Secretary of Veterans Affairs Robert Wilkie. Its total membership eventually reached 27 administration officials. Some critics claimed that the group lacked a clear leadership structure and a specific focus, which prevented it from making rapid, informed decisions to curtail the spread of SARS-CoV-2.

On March 16, Trump began conducting the daily task force press briefings at the White House. By this time, the United States had logged more than 4,000 confirmed COVID-19 cases and 70 deaths. Some public health experts warned that without immediate, drastic intervention, the nation appeared to be on a trajectory to experience an explosion of cases like the one that occurred in Italy, where hospitals became overwhelmed and doctors were forced to ration scarce ventilators and life-saving care among patients. Although Trump had told worried Americans to "relax" only one day earlier, his tone changed significantly as he took the podium in the briefing room and compared the effort to contain the coronavirus outbreak to a war. "We have an invisible enemy," he stated. "This is a bad one. This is a very bad one" (McCaskill, Kenen, and Cancryn 2020).

For the first time, the president acknowledged the severity of the global pandemic, admitted that the United States did not have the virus under control, and conceded that the economic consequences could be dire. Trump recommended that the American people take dramatic action to slow the spread of SARS-CoV-2 before the number of cases overwhelmed U.S. hospitals and medical personnel. He issued new guidelines for personal behavior that included canceling gatherings of more than ten people, avoiding crowded bars and restaurants, working from home if possible, moving schoolwork online, and self-quarantining at home for anyone who experienced even minor symptoms. "Each and every one of us has a critical role to play in stopping the spread and transmission of the virus," Trump said. "If everyone makes this change or these critical changes and sacrifices now, we will rally together as one nation, and we will defeat the virus, and we're going to have a big celebration altogether. With several weeks of focused action, we can turn the corner and turn it quickly" (McCaskill, Kenen, and Cancryn 2020).

Following his remarks, Trump turned the podium over to members of the coronavirus task force. Fauci, one of the world's leading infectious disease experts, explained how the time lag between conducting tests and reporting results often led to overly optimistic views of the success of containment efforts, which made drastic changes like those suggested by the president seem unnecessary. "When you're dealing with an emerging infectious disease outbreak, you are always behind where you think you are if you think that today reflects where you really are," he stated. "Therefore, it will always seem that the best way to address it would be to be doing something that looks like it might be an overreaction. It isn't an overreaction" (McCaskill, Kenen, and Cancryn 2020).

Birx spoke about the need for Americans to adopt a community approach to combat the novel coronavirus. Although most severe and fatal cases of COVID-19 occurred among middle-aged and elderly people, she noted that young people played a key role in preventing the spread of SARS-CoV-2.

Since some young people did not experience symptoms, they could transmit the virus to vulnerable individuals without realizing it. Birx urged members of the millennial generation to take social-distancing guidelines seriously. "Public health people like myself don't always come out with compelling and exciting messages that a 25- to 35-year-old may find interesting and something that they'll take to heart," she acknowledged. "But millennials can speak to one another about how important it is in this moment to protect all of the people" (McCaskill, Kenen, and Cancryn 2020).

Trump Dominates Press Briefings

Trump continued to appear at the daily press briefings for the next six weeks, accompanied by various members of the White House Coronavirus Task Force. A *Washington Post* analysis found that the president dominated these events, speaking for more than 28 hours—or about 60 percent of the time—during the 35 briefings held between March 16 and April 24. Pence and Birx each spoke for less than 6 hours, while Fauci only spoke for 2 hours. In addition to providing updates on COVID-19 cases and information to protect public health, Trump often discussed topics unrelated to the pandemic. He frequently used the platform offered by the press briefings to praise his administration's performance, attack his political rivals, argue with members of the media, and contradict statements made by medical experts. "The briefings have come to replace Trump's campaign rallies—now on pause during the global contagion— and fulfill the president's needs and impulses in the way his arena-shaking campaign events once did: a chance for him to riff, free-associate, spar with the media, and occupy center stage," Philip Bump and Ashley Parker wrote in the *Washington Post* (2020).

In examining Trump's 13 hours of airtime during the three weeks of press conferences between April 6 and April 24, the analysts found that he spent 2 hours attacking Democrats, the media, the nation's governors, or China. He also spent 45 minutes praising himself or his administration, which included playing three propaganda-style videos touting his coronavirus response. Meanwhile, Trump devoted just over 4 minutes to expressions of concern or sympathy for victims of COVID-19—even as the U.S. death toll surpassed 40,000. Nearly one-fourth of the president's statements included false or inaccurate information, according to the analysts, amounting to 47 minutes (Bump and Parker 2020). Trump dismissed the report on Twitter, describing the *Washington Post* as "one of the worst in the 'news' business. Total slime balls!" (Pesce 2020).

Although many presidents have used the media to broadcast important messages to the American people in times of crisis, critics charged that Trump's daily appearances at the task force press conferences often resembled campaign events rather than news briefings. Supporters noted that the extensive airtime gave the president free publicity during an election year and allowed him to showcase his leadership. "Everybody in the country is talking about one thing, and it happens to be the one thing that Donald Trump is the dominant player in, and he's leading that conversation," said former White House aide Cliff Sims. "Even visually, you still have Trump on your TV screen, in front of the White House logo in the briefing room, flanked by his advisers. And then you have [Democratic presidential candidate] Joe Biden very small on your computer screen, having a Zoom conversation with [former Democratic vice president] Al Gore" (Bump and Parker 2020).

Given Trump's tendency to focus on subjects other than the coronavirus, however, some observers on both sides of the partisan divide questioned whether it was appropriate for the media to provide a daily platform for his political remarks. Yet other observers claimed that the president's appearances offered valuable insights for voters. "Now that the president himself is answering questions on a near-daily basis, we're getting exactly what we want: a window into the president's mind, transmitted directly from the president's mouth and into our microphones," Olivia Nuzzi wrote in *New York Magazine*. "It's pure access to his thoughts and ideas and emotional state, presented to the world in real time. Trump's presence at the briefings is not valuable if what we hope to get from them is factual information about the pandemic. But if we want to learn more about what the government is doing, and why it's doing what it's doing, what could be better than this?" (Nuzzi 2020).

Some political analysts predicted that giving voters such a detailed, close-up look at Trump's handling of the pandemic would ultimately prove harmful to the president's reelection bid. As the number of COVID-19 cases climbed, Biden's campaign and various progressive groups took optimistic statements from Trump's coronavirus briefings and turned them into attack ads. "It's much different to process these press conferences when the coverage before and after is the unprecedented number of people dying, the fact that we don't have tests," said Guy Cecil, chairman of a Democratic political action committee. "Long term, it is hurting the president because people can see with their own eyes and what they are feeling in their own communities what the consequences are" (Bump and Parker 2020).

Some critics argued that Trump's dominant role in the task force briefings distracted from the goal of providing medically accurate information and public health guidance to help the American people pull together and adopt measures to combat the coronavirus. "When a person turns on the television and sees the president of the United States giving inaccurately optimistic assessments of the progress of testing, vaccine research, and treatment it encourages people to be less careful with their hand-washing and social distancing than they otherwise might be. That costs lives," wrote Matthew Yglesias for Vox. "What's called for is news coverage that incorporates the fact that the president is saying things, but that focuses on providing people with accurate information" (Yglesias 2020).

The Task Force Suspends Briefings

On several occasions, Trump expressed opinions that contradicted statements made by medical experts serving on the coronavirus task force. He asserted that the number of COVID-19 cases was declining when statistics indicated otherwise, for instance, and he insisted that scientists were on the verge of developing an effective vaccine when experts said the process would take 12 to 18 months. Trump also claimed that coronavirus testing was widely available when many parts of the country lacked access to testing materials, and he urged governors to reopen state economies despite public health officials advising against it. The president argued with reporters who pointed out such inconsistencies and rebuffed attempts by Fauci, Birx, and other task force members to correct misinformation. Critics charged that the press briefings thus ended up sending mixed messages that sowed confusion regarding the best practices to protect public health, such as wearing masks and social distancing. "Due to the coronavirus pandemic, Americans are being asked to make sacrifices," German Lopez wrote for Vox. "It's during these kinds of times, experts say, that people need leaders to provide clear guidance" (Lopez 2020).

In one exchange, Trump questioned Fauci's assessment of the usefulness of specific drugs for treating COVID-19. A reporter inquired about whether hydroxychloroquine and chloroquine—immunosuppressant drugs commonly prescribed for arthritis that also showed promise in treating malaria—could help patients infected with the coronavirus. Fauci noted that there was little medical evidence to support the drugs' effectiveness for COVID-19. "The information that you are referring to specifically is anecdotal—it was not done in a controlled clinical trial—so you really can't make any definitive statement about it," the doctor stated. "We're trying to strike a balance between making something with a potential of an effect to the American people available. At the same time, we do it under the auspices of a protocol that would give us the information to determine if it's truly safe and effective" (Lopez 2020).

Trump then stepped to the microphone, disagreed with Fauci's cautious statement, and actively promoted using the drugs to treat COVID-19 patients. "I'm probably more of a fan of that—maybe than anybody," he said. "I'm a big fan, and we'll see what happens. We all understand what the doctor said is 100 percent correct: It's early. But I have seen things that are impressive. We'll see. We're gonna know soon." Trump repeated his support for the drugs in response to further questions, although he did not offer any scientific evidence to back his opinion. "I feel good about it. That's all it is: Just a feeling. I'm a smart guy," he said. "I've been right a lot. Let's see what happens" (Lopez 2020).

On April 23, the daily briefing featured a presentation by Bill Bryan, head of the Science and Technology Directorate at the Department of Homeland Security. Bryan outlined the results of research showing that both ultraviolet light and chemical disinfectants reduced the amount of time SARS-CoV-2 virus particles remained alive on surfaces. After the presentation concluded, Trump took the podium and responded with what *Atlantic* writer Andrew Ferguson called "an instant landmark in the history of presidential utterance" (Ferguson 2020). The president mused aloud about applying that knowledge to treat COVID-19 infections inside the human body. "So, supposing we hit the body with a tremendous— whether it's ultraviolet or just very powerful light—and I think you said that hasn't been checked, but you're going to test it. And then I said supposing you brought the light inside the body, which you can do either through the skin or in some other way," Trump said. "And then I see the disinfectant, where it knocks it out in one minute. And is there a way we can do something like that by injection inside or almost a cleaning? Because you see it gets in the lungs and it does a tremendous number on the lungs, so it'd be interesting to check that" (Fottrell 2020).

Trump's comments drew widespread criticism from health care professionals, who expressed concern that people might inject disinfectants in a misguided and hazardous attempt to kill the coronavirus. "This notion of injecting or ingesting any type of cleansing product into the body is irresponsible and it's dangerous," said global health policy expert Vin Gupta. "It's a common method that people utilize when they want to kill themselves" (Fottrell 2020). The manufacturer of Lysol, Reckitt Benckiser, issued a statement disavowing Trump's comments and warning consumers against administering its products into the human body. "Our disinfectant and hygiene products should only be used as intended and in line with usage guidelines," it said. "We have a responsibility in providing consumers with access to accurate, up-to-date information as advised by leading public health experts" (Fottrell 2020).

Trump responded angrily to the controversy. He blamed the media for taking his remarks out of context and threatened to end the daily press briefings. "What is the purpose of having White House News Conferences when the Lamestream Media asks nothing but hostile questions, & then refuses to report the truth or facts accurately," he wrote on Twitter. "They get record ratings, & the American people get nothing but Fake News. Not worth the time & effort!" (Lopez 2020). On April 25, the task force canceled its daily briefing for the first time in six weeks. Over the next few days, Trump defended his comments by claiming that he intended for them to serve as a sarcastic rebuttal to what he viewed as aggressive and unfair questions by reporters. "It was said sarcastically," he declared. "It was put in the form of a question to a group of extraordinary hostile people. Namely, the fake news media" (Fottrell 2020). On May 15, the White House Coronavirus Task Force added several new members and shifted its emphasis toward formulating plans for reopening the U.S. economy. The group met infrequently, however, and did not hold further press briefings until late June, when Trump did not participate.

Further Reading

Bump, Philip, and Ashley Parker. 2020. "13 Hours of Trump." *Washington Post,* April 26, 2020. https://www.washingtonpost.com/politics/13-hours-of-trump-the-president-fills-briefings-with-attacks-and-boasts-but-little-empathy/2020/04/25/7eec5ab0-8590-11ea-a3eb-e9fc93160703_story.html.

Ferguson, Andrew. 2020. "Trump's 5 O'Clock Follies." *Atlantic,* April 25, 2020. https://www.theatlantic.com/ideas/archive/2020/04/trumps-5-oclock-follies/610717/.

Fottrell, Quentin. 2020. "Trump Floats Idea of Disinfectant for Coronavirus." MarketWatch, April 24, 2020. https://www.marketwatch.com/story/trump-suggests-disinfectant-as-treatment-for-coronavirus-by-injection-inside-or-almost-a-cleaning-doctors-call-the-idea-dangerous-2020-04-24?mod=article_inline.

Graham, David A. 2020. "Why Trump Just Can't Quit His Daily Press Conferences." *Atlantic,* April 27, 2020. https://www.theatlantic.com/ideas/archive/2020/04/end-trumps-coronavirus-briefing/610771/.

Lopez, German. 2020. "Trump's Expert Urged Caution about a Coronavirus Treatment. Trump Hyped It Up Anyway." Vox, March 20, 2020. https://www.vox.com/policy-and-politics/2020/3/20/21188397/coronavirus-trump-press-briefing-covid-19-anthony-fauci.

McCaskill, Nolan D., Joanne Kenen, and Adam Cancryn. 2020. "'This Is a Very Bad One': Trump Issues New Guidelines to Stem Coronavirus Spread." Politico, March 16, 2020. https://www.politico.com/news/2020/03/16 /trump-recommends-avoiding-gatherings-of-more-than-10-people-132323.

Nichols, Tom. 2020. "With Each Briefing, Trump Is Making Us Worse People." *Atlantic,* April 11, 2020. https://www.theatlantic.com/ideas/archive/2020 /04/each-briefing-trump-making-us-worse-people/609859/.

Nuzzi, Olivia. 2020. "The American People Should See Trump's Coronavirus Briefings in Their Entirety." *New York,* April 26, 2020. https://nymag.com /intelligencer/2020/04/trumps-coronavirus-briefings-should-be-seen-in -full.html.

Pesce, Nicole Lyn. 2020. "Three Weeks of Trump Coronavirus Briefings under a Microscope." MarketWatch, April 27, 2020. https://www.marketwatch.com /story/three-weeks-of-trump-coronavirus-briefings-under-a-microscope -2-hours-spent-on-attacks-45-minutes-on-self-congratulation-and-412 -minutes-of-condolences-for-victims-2020-04-27.

Santucci, Jeanine. 2020. "What We Know about the Coronavirus Task Force Now That Mike Pence Is in Charge." *USA Today,* February 27, 2020. https://www.usatoday.com/story/news/politics/2020/02/27/coronavirus -what-we-know-mike-pence-and-task-force/4891905002/.

Yglesias, Matthew. 2020. "Cable News Should Cancel the Trump Show." Vox, March 23, 2020. https://www.vox.com/2020/3/23/21190362/trump-daily -coronavirus-briefing-fox-cnn-msnbc.

States Issue Stay-at-Home Orders (March 19, 2020)

After the United States confirmed its first COVID-19 case on January 20, 2020, new cases appeared daily in cities across the country. Although the Donald Trump administration banned foreign nationals entering from China on January 31 and from Europe on March 11, these measures failed to prevent the novel coronavirus from gaining a foothold in the United States and spreading within the community. By mid-February, an email discussion among infectious disease experts hosted by Duane C. Caneva, chief medical officer of the U.S. Department of Homeland Security (DHS), concluded that containment of the virus was no longer feasible. Several high-ranking health officials raised the alarm and urged the federal government to launch immediate measures to mitigate the impending public health crisis (Kroll 2020).

Mitigation efforts did not commence for another month, however, and they consisted of a hodgepodge of local or regional restrictions initiated by state governors, municipal mayors, and county health departments rather than a nationwide response led by the U.S. Centers for Disease

Control and Prevention (CDC), the Federal Emergency Management Agency (FEMA), the White House Coronavirus Task Force, or other federal agencies. By the time California Governor Gavin Newsom issued the first statewide mandatory stay-at-home order on March 19, the United States had recorded nearly 14,000 COVID-19 cases. Meanwhile, Trump downplayed the threat posed by the virus, claimed that his administration had the situation under control, and resisted mitigation measures that could have a negative impact on the U.S. economy. "The challenge for the governors is there has been almost no federal guidance," said former DHS official Juliette Kayyem, "so they each have become presidents unto themselves for their own jurisdictions" (Rosenhall 2020).

States Respond to the COVID-19 Crisis

After the first known COVID-19 case appeared in Washington State, several more cases emerged on the West Coast in California and Oregon. Cities that serve as major airline hubs, such as Chicago and Boston, experienced early outbreaks as well. New York City recorded its first case on March 1 and quickly developed into a hot spot with sustained community transmission. In the absence of a coordinated federal response, some jurisdictions began implementing their own measures designed to slow the spread of the SARS-CoV-2 virus. On March 4, for instance, officials in King County, Washington—which encompasses Seattle and contains a population of 2.25 million people—issued social-distancing guidelines that recommended canceling large public events and allowing employees to telecommute if possible. Two days later, the city of San Francisco issued similar guidelines and urged vulnerable groups—such as elderly people and people with underlying health conditions—to stay at home.

At the state level, most governors declared a state of emergency or a public health emergency, which gave them broad authority to issue orders, activate personnel, access funds, and adjust regulations as needed to address a crisis. Ohio Governor Mike DeWine (R) declared a state of emergency on March 9, when his state confirmed its first COVID-19 case. Three days later, after the World Health Organization (WHO) officially designated the novel coronavirus as a global pandemic, DeWine became the first governor in the country to announce the statewide closure of public schools. Several other states immediately followed suit, while many colleges and universities across the nation suspended in-person classes and transitioned to online instruction. Although critics decried school closures as an overreaction—especially since children appeared to be less vulnerable to SARS-CoV-2 than adults—DeWine defended his decision as necessary to contain the virus. "Every day we delay, more people will die," he stated. "If we do not act and get some distance between people, our health care system in Ohio will not hold up" (Axios 2020).

On March 13, Trump declared a national emergency, which gave the states access to $50 billion in federal funds to help combat the coronavirus. At the press conference announcing the measure, however, the president flouted social-distancing rules by crowding the stage with medical experts and business executives, repeatedly touching the microphone, and shaking hands with other speakers. When reporters asked Trump about problems that had occurred in his administration's COVID-19 response—such as the failure to perform adequate testing—he declared, "I don't take responsibility at all" (Benen 2020). Trump also announced plans to increase access to coronavirus testing by establishing drive-through test sites at pharmacies nationwide.

On March 16—by which time the total number of COVID-19 cases in the United States had surpassed 5,000—the Trump administration announced a 15-day plan to "slow the spread," which included many of the same guidelines already issued by states and cities. Trump encouraged the American people to limit discretionary travel, for instance, and to avoid social gatherings of more than ten people. The guidelines took the form of recommendations rather than mandatory restrictions, and they did not include any type of national guidance for Americans to stay at home. That same day, however, six counties in the San Francisco Bay area issued mandatory shelter-in-place orders for their combined population of 6.7 million people—closing all nonessential businesses and asking residents to remain at home.

With the approach of St. Patrick's Day on March 17, many states ordered a temporary shutdown of all bars, restaurants, and nightclubs to prevent people from congregating in groups in violation of social-distancing guidelines. California, Florida, Illinois, Massachusetts, Michigan, New York, North Carolina, Ohio, Pennsylvania, and Washington all issued orders requiring bars and restaurants to close, although some allowed food service to continue on a drive-through or carryout basis. Some states went further and shut down other entertainment and recreational facilities, such as movie theaters, bowling alleys, fitness centers, casinos, wineries, museums, and water parks. Illinois Governor J.B. Pritzker (D) asserted that the strict measures became necessary when residents ignored more lenient social-distancing recommendations. "I tried earlier this week to appeal to everyone's good judgment to stay home, to avoid bars, not to congregate in crowds," he stated. "It's unfortunate that many people didn't take that seriously. The time for persuasion and public appeals is over.

The time for action is here. This is not a joke. No one is immune to this, and you have an obligation to act in the best interests of all the people in this state" (Axios 2020).

California Issues First Statewide Stay-at-Home Order

On March 19, California Governor Gavin Newsom (D) announced the nation's first statewide, mandatory stay-at-home order. Newsom's action represented the last and most drastic in a series of measures he gradually introduced to combat the spread of the coronavirus among California's 40 million residents. He initially issued guidelines limiting the size of social gatherings, then he recommended temporary closures of restaurants and schools. Newsom also convinced Disneyland to suspend its operations voluntarily. Supporters argued that the incremental approach gave residents time to adjust to the unprecedented situation, understand the value of social distancing, and accept the sacrifices necessary to address the public health crisis. "If the first we hear about it is it's a demand by the government, people tend to be less responsive," said state senator Richard Pan (D-Sacramento), a practicing physician. "We need to bring people along and have people own that decision and understand, 'This is why this is so important'" (Rosenhall 2020).

California's statewide restrictions also generated criticism, however. Opponents charged that Newsom's order went too far by closing all non-essential businesses across the state and requiring people to stay home except to buy food or exercise outdoors. They claimed that these measures would devastate the state's economy and place undue stress on households. Critics also argued that a uniform, statewide mandate was inappropriate and unnecessary given California's size and diversity. Newsom responded by emphasizing the need for caution to avoid a surge in COVID-19 cases that would exceed the capacity of the state's health care system. "We will look back at these kinds of decisions as pivotal decisions," he said. "If we're to be criticized at this moment, let us be criticized for taking this moment seriously. Let us be criticized for going full force and meeting the virus head-on" (Rosenhal 2020).

Over the next week, more than a dozen states enacted similar stay-at-home orders to slow community transmission of the coronavirus. Illinois and New Jersey adopted such measures on March 21, followed by New York on March 22, and Connecticut, Louisiana, Ohio, Oregon, and Washington on March 23. By March 28, more than half of all U.S. states and territories operated under some form of quarantine, shelter-in-place, or lockdown rules. Yet the piecemeal, state-by-state approach often created confusion among residents and caused concern among public health experts. Some contiguous states, such as North Carolina and South Carolina, adopted opposing policies. In other states, governors refused to issue statewide mandates and left it up to local officials to decide whether to establish social-distancing requirements. "With conflicting messages from the federal government and a lack of clear guidelines, states have not been on the same page, and implementation has been scattershot at best," noted a Kaiser Family Foundation assessment. "It's hard to see how a highly infectious virus is going to pay very close attention to different policies across states, let alone within them" (Kates, Michaud, and Tolbert 2020).

On March 29, Trump announced his intention to extend the federal social-distancing guidelines—originally set to expire March 31—through April 30. A week earlier, the president had predicted that the restrictions would be lifted and the country would be back to normal in time to celebrate Easter on April 12. "We had an aspiration of Easter but when you hear these kinds of numbers and you hear the potential travesty, we don't want to have a spike up," Trump explained. "Nothing would be worse than declaring victory before the victory is won" (Cummings 2020). The extension prompted several additional states to issue stay-at-home orders which, at their peak, affected 90 percent of the U.S. population. Nevertheless, critics questioned whether the lack of a coordinated, nationwide approach to mitigation might allow community spread to continue. "We are engaged in a 'natural experiment' of differing approaches to the epidemic on a massive scale," noted the Kaiser Family Foundation analysts, "and we are likely to see over the coming weeks what the consequences of that will be" (Kates, Michaud, and Tolbert 2020).

Despite the widespread implementation of stay-at-home orders by governors and mayors, the number of cases of COVID-19 in the United States increased exponentially in late March and April. On March 28, the nation exceeded 100,000 confirmed cases to surpass China and Italy as the most infected country in the world. The United States went on to reach 200,000 cases on April 1, 500,000 on April 11, and 1 million—or around one-third of the world's total cases—on April 28 (Coronavirus Research Center 2020).

Trump noted that he viewed the federal government's role in the pandemic response as providing "backup" to the states. Under the federalist system of government, the states maintained significant authority to make decisions within their borders. Yet a poll conducted by the Kaiser Family Foundation found that 60 percent of respondents wanted the federal government to take charge, while only 32 percent wanted the states to assume the primary responsibility. "The public seems to believe that in a health crisis of this magnitude, with a virus that doesn't stop at state or international borders and the death toll mounting, a more uniform and aggressive national response is needed," wrote analyst Drew Altman (2020). Dr. Anthony Fauci, the nation's leading infectious disease expert, expressed support for even stronger action to halt the pandemic. "I think we should be overly aggressive and get criticized for overreacting," he said. "I think Americans should be prepared that they are going to have to hunker down significantly more than we as a country are doing" (Axios 2020).

Further Reading

Altman, Drew. 2020. "Public Wants Federal Government, Not States, in Charge on Coronavirus." Axios, April 7, 2020. https://www.axios.com/states -federal-government-coronavirus-trump-b999862d-3e08-46f4-8707 -d9d6ab213671.html.

Axios. 2020. "States Order Bars and Restaurants to Close Due to Coronavirus." March 17, 2020. https://www.axios.com/ohio-governor-bars-restaurants -coronavirus-26e4b6e3-7f65-4f6a-abf9-f3940220cc6f.html.

Benen, Steve. 2020. "On Virus Missteps, Trump Declares, 'I Don't Take Responsibility at All.'" MSNBC, March 16, 2020. https://www.msnbc.com/rachel -maddow-show/virus-missteps-trump-declares-i-don-t-take-responsibility -all-n1160236.

Coronavirus Research Center. 2020. Johns Hopkins University. https://corona virus.jhu.edu/us-map.

Cummings, William. 2020. "Trump: Coronavirus Guidelines, Set to Expire Tuesday, Will Be Extended to April 30." *USA Today,* March 29, 2020. https://www.usatoday.com/story/news/politics/2020/03/29/coronavirus -response-updates-pelosi-fauci/2935369001/.

Kates, Jennifer, Josh Michaud, and Jennifer Tolbert. 2020. "Stay-at-Home Orders to Fight COVID-19 in the United States: The Risks of a Scattershot Approach." Kaiser Family Foundation, April 5, 2020. https://www.kff.org /coronavirus-policy-watch/stay-at-home-orders-to-fight-covid19/.

Rosenhall, Laurel. 2020. "Governor Gavin Newsom Just Slow-Walked California into a Mass Retreat from a Virus. How?" CalMatters, March 20, 2020. https://calmatters.org/politics/2020/03/gavin-newsom-california-corona virus-shutdown-order/.

Tensions Rise between Trump and Governors (March 20–April 30, 2020)

Beginning with California on March 19, 2020, most states issued stay-at-home orders in response to the COVID-19 pandemic. These orders closed nonessential businesses and required residents to shelter in place except for brief outings to obtain food or medicine. The governors who issued stay-at-home orders argued that such drastic measures were needed to slow the spread of the novel coronavirus SARS-CoV-2, which had proven highly transmissible from person to person. Officials sought to "flatten the curve," or reduce the infection rate to a level that would not exceed the capacity of hospitals and the availability of medical equipment. "In the biggest crisis of our lifetimes, governors were on the front lines and taking charge," said Maryland Governor Larry Hogan (R), chairman of the National Governors Association. "States had to make decisions and use their powers in a way I don't ever remember in my lifetime" (Balz 2020).

In such hard-hit states as California, Michigan, New York, and Washington, governors pleaded for federal assistance in acquiring the resources they needed to manage the public health crisis, such as ventilators for severely ill patients, personal protective equipment (PPE) for first responders, test kits to identify carriers of the virus, and funding to help pay for it. Some governors expressed frustration with President Donald Trump and criticized what they viewed as a lack of federal leadership and coordination. Trump responded by claiming that the states had everything they should need, blaming the governors for mishandling the crisis, and dismissing the complaints as politically motivated.

Tensions rose in April as the virtual shutdown in the operations of most states caused mass unemployment and economic hardship nationwide. Trump increasingly asserted his authority and pressured states to reopen, but some governors resisted, saying that it was not yet safe to do so. Critics charged that the president's support for efforts to "liberate" citizens from state lockdowns undermined the shared sense of national responsibility and sacrifice necessary to combat the coronavirus. "There was no leadership from Washington," said Illinois Governor J. B. Pritzker (D). "Is it hard to do? Sure. But it's part of the job. That's what leadership is. Leadership is stepping out front and showing people the direction they need to go that they don't necessarily understand or agree with" (Balz 2020).

Governors Request Federal Assistance

As COVID-19 cases appeared across the United States in February and early March, many state and local officials began implementing strategies to mitigate the spread of the virus. By March 28, when the number of confirmed cases nationwide exceeded 100,000, more than half of all U.S. states and territories operated under some form of stay-at-home, shelter-in-place, or lockdown rules to limit contact between residents. In the hardest-hit areas, such as New York City, the steep rise in cases overwhelmed hospitals and caused shortages of critical medical supplies. A number of governors and mayors requested urgent assistance from the federal government to acquire masks, gowns, ventilators, and other materials.

Trump responded to some of the requests for medical equipment by telling the governors to "try getting it yourselves" (Alexander 2020). He also blamed the shortages on his predecessor, President Barack Obama, claiming that the former administration had failed to stockpile sufficient quantities of ventilators and other equipment to prepare for the crisis. Members of the Obama administration disagreed, arguing that the national stockpile was only intended to serve as a stopgap measure until the federal government could purchase or manufacture needed supplies. On March 18, Trump invoked the Defense Production Act, which gave him the authority to enlist U.S. industries in producing vital equipment to address a national emergency. Yet he also expressed reluctance to use this authority to help the states. "The federal government is not supposed to be out there buying vast amounts of items and then shipping," the president said. "You know, we're not a shipping clerk" (Balz 2020).

Without federal intervention, the states ended up competing against one another to purchase the necessary items at significant markups. "What we're doing is creating a world of winners and losers rather than accounting for priorities based on timings, needs, and best use," said Steve Schooner, a government procurement expert from George Washington University (Kroll 2020). Some governors improvised ways to acquire much-needed supplies. Massachusetts Governor Charlie Baker (R), for instance, managed to purchase 1.2 million N95 masks from China and borrowed the New England Patriots' team plane to transport them to Boston. Critics expressed outrage that the states had to go to such lengths and asserted that the federal government abdicated its responsibility to coordinate the supply chain. "It is dangerous on the granular level not to have the federal government use its unique powers and resources to deliver goods and services that they can uniquely do, and that they can get the best price for. And do it in a fair and transparent manner," said Kathleen Sebelius, former secretary of Health and Human Services. "There's no question it's costing lives" (Knotts and Chakrabarti 2020).

Trump lashed out publicly at several governors who criticized his administration's response. As New York emerged as the epicenter of the U.S. coronavirus outbreak, the president complained that Governor Andrew Cuomo (D) was "calling daily, even hourly, begging for everything, most of which should have been the state's responsibility, such as new hospitals, beds, ventilators, etc. I got it all done for him" (Smith 2020). Trump questioned whether New York truly needed additional ventilators and accused Cuomo of mismanaging available supplies. When Washington Governor Jay Inslee (D) suggested that state efforts to combat SARS-CoV-2 would be more effective if the Trump administration "stuck to the science and told the truth," the president called Inslee a "snake" and told Vice President Mike Pence not to deal with him (Choi 2020). "To be gracious, part of it is the fog of war. It's people having to do 50 things in five minutes," Inslee said in explaining the terse exchange. "But it is no secret that the president did not have the intense focus he needed in the first month of this" (Balz 2020).

Trump became embroiled in another public dispute with Michigan Governor Gretchen Whitmer (D). When Michigan emerged as a coronavirus hot spot, Whitmer expressed frustration with what she viewed as a lack of "clear and concise guidance from the federal government." Trump responded by saying that "I don't know if she knows what's going on, but all she does is sit there and blame the federal government" (Soicher 2020). The president also referred to the governor dismissively as "the woman in Michigan" and "Gretchen 'Half' Whitmer" (Alexander 2020) and claimed that she went overboard by restricting the sale of home improvement and gardening materials as part of her social-distancing guidelines. "She has things—don't buy paint, don't buy roses—I mean she's got all these crazy things," Trump stated. "Some of them are being unreasonable" (Reston 2020). Supporters noted that each state faced unique circumstances that required governors to remain flexible and tailor their responses to local conditions.

Trump accused Democrats of sowing division in a time of national crisis and politicizing the coronavirus in an effort to harm his 2020 reelection bid. On several occasions, Trump threatened to withhold federal assistance unless governors praised his administration's response to the pandemic. "If they don't treat you right, I don't call," he declared (Alexander 2020). Critics argued that the coronavirus did not respect state borders, so the federal government ultimately bore responsibility for protecting the American people. "We need two things from the federal government. We need help on that supply chain, especially when it becomes international, and we need coordination and basic partnership," Cuomo stated. "When you fund the state government, you just are funding a state government to perform the functions you want us to perform" (Reston 2020).

Disputes over Testing Capacity

Within a few weeks, as the dire economic impact of the state shutdowns became clear and the American people grew increasingly weary of staying at home, Trump began pressuring the nation's governors to lift restrictions and return to normal. Although reopening businesses held strong appeal for people struggling with unemployment and financial hardship, the governors faced a difficult tradeoff between protecting residents' health and restoring their states' economic base. "The worst scenario," Cuomo explained, "would be if we did all of this, we got that number [of cases] down, everybody went to extraordinary means, and then we go to reopen and we reopen too fast or we reopen and there's unanticipated consequences, and we see that number go up again" (Smith 2020).

Many governors resisted the pressure to reopen, arguing that they could not do so safely without much greater testing capability. They noted that fast, accurate, and extensive coronavirus testing would enable state officials to identify and isolate new cases, trace contacts and apply selective quarantine measures, monitor infection rates, and contain new outbreaks. As public health experts pointed out, the countries that had reopened successfully employed aggressive, nationwide testing regimens to halt the spread of SARS-CoV-2. "These things were done in Germany, in Italy, in Greece, Vietnam, in Singapore, in New Zealand, and in China," said federal health care adviser Andy Slavitt. "They were not secret. . . . Not mysterious. And these were not all wealthy countries. They just took accountability for getting it done. But we did not do that here" (Shear et al. 2020).

The original COVID-19 test process developed by the U.S. Centers for Disease Control and Prevention (CDC) involved inserting a nasopharyngeal swab (a long plastic swab with a foam tip) into the nose and collecting a sample from deep inside the patient's sinus cavity. The sample was placed in a sterile vial filled with Viral Transport Medium (VTM) and sent to a laboratory, where a chemical reagent was used to detect the presence of SARS-CoV-2. During the early months of the coronavirus outbreak in the United States, the test kits distributed by the CDC contained a nonfunctioning ingredient and produced faulty results. In addition, the U.S. Food and Drug Administration initially refused to allow independent laboratories to develop or process tests, which contributed to backlogs and delays.

Although U.S. testing capacity improved in April, many states still experienced shortages of test kits and related equipment, such as swabs, reagents, masks, and laboratory facilities to process the tests. Former CDC director Tom Frieden asserted that the 150,000 daily tests being conducted nationwide in mid-April needed to increase tenfold for any hope of containment. "We really need the federal government, commercial laboratories, private sector hospitals to continue to step up," he stated. "The federal government has a crucial role to play in ensuring the supply chain here and focusing on ramping up test capacity" (Reston 2020).

Several governors complained about the limited availability of testing materials and warned that they could not safely reopen their states without resolving the issue. "We need more swabs, we've been very direct and pointed in terms of working with our partners at FEMA [the Federal Emergency Management Agency] to try to procure those swabs," said California Governor Gavin Newsom (D). "We could be doing exponentially more [testing]. We'll be looking for all the support we can get—private, public, federal, local, state." Ohio Governor Mike DeWine (R) claimed that his state could double or triple its testing capacity with greater access to reagent chemicals. "It's a supply chain production problem and that's really what is holding it back," he stated. "We have a shortage, worldwide shortage, of some of the materials that go into this. So, we really need help" (Reston 2020).

Trump responded indignantly to suggestions that his administration failed to provide adequate testing materials. He argued that the governors exaggerated the problem to negatively shape public opinion of his coronavirus response. The president asserted that the states could be conducting an additional one million tests per week if they took advantage of the available capacity. "We have tremendous capacity," he declared. "The governors know that. The Democrat governors know that. They're the ones that are complaining" (Reston 2020). Trump also said that his administration planned to send 5.5 million more swabs to the states, even though acquiring such materials "can be done easily by the governors themselves. Mostly it's cotton. It's not a big deal, you can get cotton easily, but if they can't get it, we will take care of it" (Reston 2020).

During an April 20 White House Coronavirus Task Force press briefing, Trump mocked Hogan's claim that Maryland needed more testing capacity. After Dr. Deborah Birx displayed a map indicating the location of laboratory facilities in the state, the president appeared incredulous that the governor "really didn't know about the federal laboratories" (Shear et al. 2020). When state officials contacted a National Institutes of Health facility marked on the map, however, they learned that it could not process COVID-19 tests due to a shortage of testing materials. "To say that the governors have plenty of testing and they should just get to work on testing—somehow we aren't doing our job—is just absolutely false,"

Hogan stated. "When the White House says there's plenty of 'testing capacity' in the states, they are referring to the number of tests that could be run on machines that exist in hospitals, commercial labs, and doctors' offices. So, why aren't states using all the capacity? There's a worldwide shortage of swabs, VTM, and reagent. Can't do tests without all of those. And they don't come in a package—you have to buy each of those from multiple suppliers" (Shesgreen and Groppe 2020).

Trump Pressures States to Reopen

Tensions between the president and the governors rose further in late April. With the federal recommendations for Americans to limit discretionary travel and avoid large gatherings set to expire on April 30, Trump applied pressure on the states to relax their social-distancing rules and allow businesses to reopen by May 1. "Once we OPEN UP OUR GREAT COUNTRY, and it will be sooner rather than later, the horror of the Invisible Enemy, except for those that sadly lost a family member or friend, must be quickly forgotten," he tweeted. "Our Economy will BOOM, perhaps like never before!!!" (Lutz 2020). Trump also controversially expressed support for anti-lockdown protests against governors who imposed strict stay-at-home orders, encouraging demonstrators to "liberate" Michigan, Minnesota, and Virginia. Meanwhile, infectious disease expert and task force member Dr. Anthony Fauci called the May 1 deadline "overly optimistic" and advised a cautious approach bolstered by an extensive testing program. "We have to have something in place that is efficient and that we can rely on, and we're not there yet," he stated (BBC News 2020).

Facing resistance to his reopening timeline, Trump insisted that he had the power to force states to end their lockdowns. "When somebody is the president of the United States, the authority is total," he declared at a press conference. Trump argued that he "calls the shots" with regard to the coronavirus response and that the governors "can't do anything without the approval of the president of the United States" (BBC News 2020). Legal experts contradicted Trump's assertions, noting that the U.S. Constitution gave the states, rather than the federal government, responsibility for maintaining public safety. Other observers pointed out that Trump's position conflicted with his earlier statements demanding that the states assume greater responsibility for fighting the pandemic. "Some of the most over-the-top claims we've seen about the relationship between federal power and state power are happening at the same time that the federal government is shockingly inactive in areas it could and should be," said law professor Robert Chesney (Balz 2020).

Some governors pushed back against Trump's pressure to reopen. "We don't have a king, we have a president," Cuomo stated. "If he says to me, 'I declare it open,' and that is a public health risk or it's reckless with the welfare of the people of my state, I will oppose it. And then we will have a constitutional crisis like you haven't seen in decades, where states tell the federal government, 'We're not going to follow your order.' It would be terrible for this country. It would be terrible for this president" (Smith 2020). Ten states joined regional pacts to coordinate their reopening plans and to present a united front in the face of Trump's demands. Cuomo led an alliance of seven East Coast states (Connecticut, Delaware, Massachusetts, New Jersey, New York, and Pennsylvania), while Newsom headed a coalition of three West Coast states (California, Oregon, and Washington).

Polls indicated that the governors enjoyed more popular support than the president when it came to handling the coronavirus. A *Washington Post*/University of Maryland survey released April 21 found that 72 percent of Americans approved of their governor's response to the crisis, while only 15 to 20 percent felt that their state's social-distancing restrictions were too tough. "[The governors] are much more on the ground, dealing with these problems, day-to-day," said public affairs expert Terry Madonna. "It could be that they're closer to the voters and therefore able to explain better to their constituents what they're doing and why they're doing it" (Shesgreen and Groppe 2020).

Some of the Democratic governors Trump criticized for overreacting to the public health threat saw their public approval ratings increase dramatically. Whitmer received a 24-point boost, for instance, as did Wisconsin Governor Tony Evers. Meanwhile, 54 percent of Americans nationwide disapproved of Trump's performance (Shesgreen and Groppe 2020). Some observers noted that public opinion played an important role in reopening the economy, because citizens had to feel safe leaving their homes, returning to work, and resuming their normal lives. "Who are they going to trust?" said political analyst Susan Del Percio. "Are they going to trust the president to say, 'Things are great, go ahead,' or are they going to trust their respective governors who have been giving them the straight facts?" (Smith 2020).

Within a few days, Trump backed away from his authoritative stance on reopening the economy and expressed willingness to let the states determine their own schedules. "I will be authorizing each individual governor, of each individual state, to implement a reopening and a very powerful reopening plan of their state in a time and a manner as most appropriate," he said. "Certain states are in [a] much different condition and in a much different place than other states. . . . The federal government will be watching them very closely and will be there to help in many different ways" (Smith 2020). Trump pledged to work in conjunction with the governors and not to exert pressure on states to reopen. The president made the reversal in his position clear by criticizing Georgia Governor Brian Kemp (R) for ignoring public health guidelines and reopening businesses in his state too quickly. "I told the governor very simply that I disagree with his decision, but he has to do what he thinks is right," Trump stated (Balz 2020).

Critics charged that the inconsistent approach taken by the White House caused confusion and uncertainty among the American people. "It's very dangerous to have mixed messages coming out of the federal government questioning everything from when we're going to open up, and who's in charge of that, to whether we have a serious disease," said Sebelius. "What that does is undermine any confidence that people are getting straight information in a very difficult time" (Knott and Chakrabarti 2020). Some critics claimed that Trump's eagerness to lift stay-at-home orders and reopen the economy weakened citizens' commitment to following state social-distancing mandates, impaired the national response, and set the stage for a resurgence of the coronavirus.

Further Reading

Alexander, Erik B. 2020. "Beating COVID-19 Demands President Trump Work With, Not Against, Governors." *Washington Post,* April 13, 2020. https://www.washingtonpost.com/outlook/2020/04/03/beating-covid-19-demands-president-trump-work-with-not-against-governors/.

Balz, Dan. 2020. "As Washington Stumbled, Governors Stepped to the Forefront." *Washington Post,* May 3, 2020. https://www.washingtonpost.com/graphics/2020/politics/power-to-states-and-governors-during-coronavirus/.

BBC News. 2020. "Coronavirus: Trump Feuds with Governors over Authority." April 14, 2020. https://www.bbc.com/news/world-us-canada-522 74969.

Choi, Matthew. 2020. "Trump Calls Inslee a 'Snake' over Criticism of Coronavirus Rhetoric." Politico, March 6, 2020. https://www.politico.com/news/2020/03/06/donald-trump-jay-inslee-coronavirus-123114.

Knotts, Brittany, and Meghna Chakrabarti. 2020. "The Role of Governors and the Federal Government during the Coronavirus Pandemic." WBUR, April 16, 2020. https://www.wbur.org/onpoint/2020/04/16/kathleen-sebelius-coronavirus-states-government.

Kroll, Andy. 2020. "'Absolute Clusterf**k': Inside the Denial and Dysfunction of Trump's Coronavirus Task Force." *Rolling Stone,* April 13, 2020. https://www.rollingstone.com/politics/politics-features/trump-coronavirus-covid-white-house-testing-kushner-cdc-dysfunction-red-dawn-982308/.

Lutz, Eric. 2020. "Trump's May 1 Coronavirus Deadline Is More Wishful Thinking." *Vanity Fair,* April 15, 2020. https://www.vanityfair.com/news/2020 /04/trump-may-1-coronavirus-deadline-more-wishful-thinking.

Reston, Maeve. 2020. "Governors Dispute Trump's Claim that There's Enough Coronavirus Testing." CNN, April 19, 2020. https://www.cnn.com/2020 /04/19/politics/trump-governors-coronavirus-testing/index.html.

Shear, Michael D., Noah Weiland, Eric Lipton, Maggie Haberman, and David E. Sanger. 2020. "Inside Trump's Failure: The Rush to Abandon Leadership Role on the Virus." *New York Times,* July 19, 2020. https://www.nytimes .com/2020/07/18/us/politics/trump-coronavirus-response-failure-leader ship.html.

Shesgreen, Deirdre, and Maureen Groppe. 2020. "Anti-Quarantine Protests, Trump Pressure Put Governors on Political Tightrope over Coronavirus." *USA Today,* April 22, 2020. https://www.usatoday.com/story/news/world /2020/04/22/coronavirus-governors-michigan-whitmer-florida-desantis -key-states-face-trump-pressure-amid-response/5169260002/.

Smith, Allan. 2020. "Trump Backs Down after Cuomo, Other Governors Unite on Coronavirus Response." NBC News, April 14, 2020. https://www .nbcnews.com/politics/donald-trump/trump-backs-down-after-cuomo -governors-unite-coronavirusk-response-n1183471.

Soicher, Spencer. 2020. "President Trump and Governor Whitmer Exchange More Jabs." WILX, March 27, 2020. https://www.wilx.com/content/news /President-Trump-and-Gov-Whitmer-569155591.html.

Congress Passes the CARES Act (March 27, 2020)

As a growing number of states imposed social-distancing measures to slow the spread of the coronavirus, economic activity in the United States ground to a halt. Business shutdowns, school closures, travel restrictions, and event cancellations resulted in unprecedented job losses, with 3.3 million Americans—almost five times more than the previous record—filing for unemployment benefits during the week ending March 21 (Phillips 2020). The U.S. Congress responded by passing the Coronavirus Aid, Relief, and Economic Security (CARES) Act, which President Donald Trump signed into law on March 27. "I just signed the CARES Act, the single biggest economic relief package in American History—twice as large as any relief bill ever enacted," Trump tweeted afterward. "At $2.2 Trillion Dollars, this bill will deliver urgently needed relief for our nation's families, workers, and businesses" (Cathey 2020). The CARES Act provided one-time economic impact payments to more than 150 million Americans, temporarily boosted unemployment compensation, and provided loans and other aid to help small businesses, large corporations, and state and local governments weather the crisis.

Economic Downturn Spurs Legislative Action

In mid-March, as the number of confirmed COVID-19 cases in the United States approached 100,000 and state after state enacted stay-at-home orders, companies across the country shuttered their operations and laid off employees. The global pandemic disrupted nearly every aspect of the U.S. economy. Demand for air travel declined precipitously, prompting the U.S. airline industry to request a $50 billion federal bailout to keep domestic carriers afloat. With consumers forced to hunker down at home, the U.S. restaurant industry predicted it would lose $225 billion and shed up to 7 million workers within three months. U.S. Secretary of the Treasury Steve Mnuchin warned that the national unemployment rate could climb above 20 percent, while the financial industry braced for a 25 percent drop in U.S. gross national product (GNP) during the second quarter of 2020. Members of Congress compared the potential magnitude of the economic disaster to the Great Depression of the 1930s. "The circumstances in which we live in now have no precedent, at least for 70 years, and even there, it's unique," said Senator Marco Rubio (R-FL). "It is a catastrophic collapse of the economy via government fiat" (Phillips 2020).

Congress enacted the first phase of its legislative response to the COVID-19 emergency on March 6 with the passage of the Coronavirus Preparedness and Response Supplemental Appropriations Act. This law allocated $8.3 billion in federal funds to public health agencies on the front lines of the crisis, including the Centers for Disease Control and Prevention (CDC), the Food and Drug Administration (FDA), the National Institutes of Health (NIH), and state and local agencies. Lawmakers earmarked the funds for promoting vaccine development, acquiring medical supplies, and increasing hospital capacity. On March 18, Congress completed a second phase of legislative activity by passing the Families First Coronavirus Response Act. This law allocated $104 billion to establish free coronavirus testing, provide paid sick and family leave for people affected by COVID-19, and increase nutrition assistance and other social welfare benefits for low-income Americans.

Over the next week, Congressional Democrats and Republicans continued meeting with Mnuchin to negotiate a larger economic stimulus package to help mitigate some of the damage caused by the coronavirus lockdowns. Some observers questioned whether the two political parties could find enough common ground to enact major relief legislation. Partisan disagreements had seemingly reached a new peak in late January and early February, when the Democratic-controlled House of Representatives voted to impeach Trump on charges of abuse of power and obstruction of Congress, and the Republican-controlled Senate voted to acquit the president and keep him in office. Yet congressional leaders—including Senate Majority Leader Mitch McConnell (R-KY), Senate Minority Leader Chuck Schumer (D-NY), Speaker of the House Nancy Pelosi (D-CA), and House Minority Leader Kevin McCarthy (R-CA)—managed to put aside their differences and craft bipartisan relief legislation. "A crisis can motivate action, not so much because it's the 'right thing to do' but because neither party wants to be blamed for failing to act," said Sarah Binder, a professor of political science at George Washington University. "When the consequences of stalemate are too steep for both parties (an economy in a coma, millions already filing for unemployment, tens of thousands dying), we shouldn't be surprised to see them go to the bargaining table and reach a deal" (Matthews 2020).

On March 25, the Senate passed the CARES Act by a unanimous 96-0 vote, with the four remaining members in self-quarantine due to coronavirus concerns. The House had four confirmed COVID-19 cases by that time as well as a dozen additional members in self-quarantine. As a result, House leaders called for a voice vote—a procedural measure that would allow members to avoid traveling to Washington, DC, to cast individually recorded votes. Instead, members who chose to remain at home could post videos on the public affairs network C-SPAN explaining their positions on the bill. Representative Thomas Massie (R-KY) objected to this plan, and he filed a motion on March 26 calling for a quorum to vote in person. Trump expressed outrage about the delay. "Workers & small businesses need money now in order to survive. Virus wasn't their fault," he tweeted. "It is 'HELL' dealing with the Dems, had to give up some stupid things in order to get the 'big picture' done. 90% GREAT! WIN BACK HOUSE, but throw Massie out of Republican Party!" (Grisales et al. 2020).

House leaders from both parties emphasized the importance of passing the legislation quickly to free up federal resources to fight the pandemic. "This is an emergency, a challenge to the conscience as well as the budget of our country, and every dollar that we spend is an investment in the lives and the livelihood of the American people," Pelosi declared. "This is not another day in Congress," McCarthy added. "This is a time when we have to come together to deliver results" (Grisales et al. 2020). The House went on to approve the CARES Act by voice vote on March 27. Although no Democrats attended the signing ceremony in the Oval Office later that day, Trump praised the bipartisan effort that culminated in the relief package. "I want to thank Democrats and Republicans for coming together and putting America first," he stated (Grisales et al. 2020).

At $2.2 trillion, the CARES Act became the largest economic stimulus package ever enacted in U.S. history. Economists estimated that it amounted to around 10 percent of the nation's gross domestic product (GDP). It exceeded the $830 billion American Recovery and Reinvestment Act, which Congress passed in 2009 in response to the Great Recession, and also surpassed the fiscal stimulus aspects of the New Deal legislation Congress passed during the 1930s to combat the Great Depression. "It's one of the most major pieces of legislation we've done," Schumer acknowledged. "The gears of the American economy have ground to a halt. Our country has faced immense challenges before, but rarely so many at the same time" (Phillips 2020). Dylan Matthews (2020) of Vox described the CARES Act as "transformative," while Amber Phillips (2020) of the *Washington Post* called it "unprecedented" and noted that its passage "underscores just how fearful lawmakers are of not acting immediately to prop up an economy that has already fallen off a cliff."

Some of the main elements of the CARES Act put money in the pockets of ordinary Americans in an effort to strengthen the social safety net and prevent families from descending into poverty during the pandemic. The legislation allocated $300 billion to provide one-time cash payments to more than 160 million people. These economic impact payments—which phased out at household incomes over $150,000 per year—amounted to $1,200 for individuals or $2,400 for married couples, plus $500 for each child under age 18. In addition, the CARES Act provided $260 billion to increase unemployment compensation by $600 per week and expand unemployment benefits to cover self-employed, freelance, contract, and gig workers. The legislation also aided families by deferring payments on federal student loans, extending deadlines for federal tax payments, and prohibiting foreclosure and eviction proceedings for 120 days.

The CARES Act also featured provisions aimed at helping American businesses that experienced financial distress due to the coronavirus lockdowns. The legislation allocated more than $500 billion in "economic stabilization funding" for large corporations—in the form of interest-free loans, tax breaks, and emergency aid—with restrictions to prevent companies from using the money for stock buybacks or executive compensation. It also provided more than $350 billion in forgivable loans for small businesses (defined as having fewer than 500 employees) through the

Paycheck Protection Program (PPP). Finally, the CARES Act provided $340 billion to help state and local governments respond to the public health crisis, as well as $150 billion to aid hospitals and health care facilities in treating COVID-19 patients. Other provisions required health insurance companies to cover coronavirus testing and related expenses and changed FDA rules to speed up the approval of vaccines and treatments.

Impact and Criticism

To ensure that the historic $2.2 trillion CARES Act funding was spent responsibly, Congress established two entities to provide oversight. The Pandemic Response Accountability Committee, comprised of inspectors general from nine different federal departments, was charged with promoting transparency and preventing fraud, waste, and mismanagement in the administration of the relief and stimulus funds. In addition, the legislation created the position of special inspector general for pandemic relief (SIGPR) to oversee distribution of the $500 billion bailout for large corporations. The legislation required the SIGPR to issue independent reports detailing which companies received loans or other taxpayer-funded benefits from the CARES Act. It also required the SIGPR to inform Congress if the White House interfered with the release of such information.

According to critics, the Trump administration took steps to undermine these oversight provisions as soon as Congress passed the CARES Act. Upon approving the legislation, Trump added a signing statement objecting to the SIGPR's powers and declaring that he would not permit the inspector general "to issue reports to the Congress without the presidential supervision" (Wilkie and Macias 2020). On March 30, members of the Pandemic Response Accountability Committee selected Glenn Fine, inspector general of the U.S. Department of Defense, to serve as its chairman. A few days later, Trump removed Fine from the post, claiming that he had received "reports of bias" about the inspector general and suggesting that Fine was a Democratic appointee (Wilkie and Macias 2020). In fact, Fine had originally been appointed by Republican president George W. Bush. Schumer issued a statement condemning the president's actions. "President Trump is abusing the coronavirus pandemic to eliminate honest and independent public servants because they are willing to speak truth to power and because he is so clearly afraid of strong oversight," he wrote. "President Trump's corrupt action to sideline [Fine] only strengthens Democrats' resolve to hold the administration accountable and enforce the multiple strict oversight provisions of the CARES Act" (Wilkie and Macias 2020).

Progressive critics charged that billions of dollars in CARES Act money were directed to large corporations and wealthy political donors who did not need federal assistance. Brookings Institution researchers Aryeh Mellman and Norman Eisen (2020) reported that lobbyists connected to the Trump administration collected more than $10 billion in relief funds on behalf of two dozen corporate clients, for instance, while another $273 million went to 100 companies owned or operated by key financial supporters of Trump's reelection campaign. The researchers also identified family members of Secretary of Transportation Elaine Chao, Secretary of Agriculture Sonny Perdue, and White House senior adviser and Trump son-in-law Jared Kushner among the major CARES Act beneficiaries. They argued that these loans created potential conflicts of interest. "The existence of vigorous oversight will ensure that the money disbursed by the CARES Act gets to the people who need and are entitled to those funds," Mellman and Eisen wrote. "Conversely, inadequate oversight will mean favorable treatment for friends of the president and less relief for struggling small business owners and other American firms and individuals."

The Paycheck Protection Program, which featured $350 billion in low-interest loans to help small businesses survive the pandemic, ran out of funds in less than two weeks. Although Mnuchin initially refused to reveal where the money went, he eventually produced a list of recipients under congressional pressure. Critics noted that billions of dollars in PPP loans flowed to companies in states that had relatively few COVID-19 cases. Businesses in Texas received more PPP funds than businesses in New York, for example, even though Texas had less than 8 percent of New York's 216,000 COVID-19 cases (Gandel 2020). In addition, firms in the construction industry claimed the largest share of PPP funds, even though most states deemed construction an essential service and allowed companies to continue regular operations. Finally, critics noted that $250 million worth of PPP loans went to publicly traded companies that had other options available for raising capital. Some of these companies—including the national restaurant chains Potbelly, Shake Shack, and Ruth's Chris Steak House—returned the money following public backlash.

Conservative critics also complained about poor administration of CARES Act funds aimed at assisting unemployed workers and their families. They pointed out that over $1 million in economic impact payments intended to supplement the income of ordinary Americans during the pandemic were issued to deceased individuals. Some of the $1,200 checks also mistakenly went to young people who were claimed as dependents on their parents' tax returns. In addition, critics described the $600 per week federal increase to regular state unemployment compensation as excessive and claimed that it created an incentive for recipients not to work. Trump and Republican lawmakers argued that unemployed people needed to return to work as soon as possible for the U.S. economy to reopen successfully. For two-thirds of unemployed workers, however, the amount they received in unemployment benefits exceeded their regular weekly salaries (Matthews 2020). Supporters of the boost in unemployment compensation, on the other hand, contended that the payments served their intended purpose by enabling workers to stay at home during state lockdowns without experiencing financial hardship. "Deterring work in this circumstance was a feature, not a bug," of the CARES Act, according to Matthews (2020).

Studies suggested that both the economic impact payments and the boost in unemployment compensation helped low- and middle-income Americans survive the coronavirus shutdowns. Although the U.S. unemployment rate more than tripled in April, from 4.4 percent to 14.7 percent, personal income grew by 10.5 percent for the month. As a result, low-income households increased their spending by 26 percent immediately following implementation of the stimulus package. According to researchers from Columbia University, the CARES Act thus bolstered consumer spending while also preventing 12 million Americans from descending into poverty (Matthews 2020). In contrast, economists found little evidence of positive impact on employment levels or business survival from the PPP small business loans or the $500 billion provided to large corporations.

After cooperating to pass the CARES Act, Democrats and Republicans disagreed about the effectiveness of various provisions and the need for additional relief and stimulus bills. Trump predicted that the CARES Act would trigger an immediate economic rebound. "We're going to keep our small businesses strong and our big businesses strong. And that's keeping our country strong and our jobs strong," he declared. "In a fairly short period of time because of what they've done and what everyone's done, I really think we're going to be stronger than ever and we'll be protected from a lot of this" (Grisales et al. 2020). Republican leaders expressed reluctance to discuss further economic measures until they could evaluate the effectiveness of the CARES Act and assess the nation's progress in fighting the coronavirus. "Let's let this bill work," McCarthy stated. "Whatever decision we have to make going forward, let's do it with knowledge, let's do [it] with experience of what's on the ground at that moment in time" (Grisales et al. 2020).

Democratic leaders, on the other hand, argued that further legislation was needed to protect working families from severe economic hardship. On May 15, the Democratic-controlled House passed the Health and

Economic Recovery Omnibus Emergency Solutions Act (HEROES Act), a $3 trillion supplemental stimulus package that proposed extending unemployment benefits through January 2021 and issuing additional economic impact checks. The Republican-controlled Senate refused to vote on the legislation. Other Democratic proposals provided monthly cash payments to all Americans for the duration of the pandemic or extended unemployment benefits until employment levels recovered to a specific threshold. Congress failed to reach agreement on any further bills, however, even as the $600 weekly unemployment boost expired on July 31. "The Trump administration and its allies in Congress appear set to follow up one of the most ambitious measures adopted in American history with absolutely nothing," Matthews wrote. "The result of that will likely be that all the progress in terms of poverty and recovered spending among the poor enabled by the CARES Act will be undone" (Matthews 2020).

Further Reading

Cathey, Libby. 2020. "Coronavirus Government Response Updates: Trump Signs $2T Relief Bill after House Passage." ABC News, March 27, 2020. https://abcnews.go.com/Politics/coronavirus-government-response -updates-drama-house-votes-2t/story?id=69833576.

Gandel, Stephen. 2020. "Paycheck Protection Program Billions Went to Large Companies and Missed Virus Hot Spots." CBS News, April 20, 2020. https://www.cbsnews.com/news/paycheck-protection-program-small -businesses-large-companies-coroanvirus/.

Grisales, Claudia, Kelsey Snell, Susan Davis, and Barbara Sprunt. 2020. "President Trump Signs $2 Trillion Coronavirus Rescue Package into Law." NPR, March 27, 2020. https://www.npr.org/2020/03/27/822062909 /house-aims-to-send-2-trillion-rescue-package-to-president-to-stem -coronavirus-cr.

Matthews, Dylan. 2020. "Congress's COVID-19 Rescue Plan Was Bigger Than the New Deal. It's about to End." Vox, July 7, 2020. https://www.vox.com /future-perfect/2020/7/7/21308450/extra-600-unemployment-stimulus -expiring-cares-act.

Melman, Aryeh, and Norman Eisen. 2020. "Addressing the Other COVID Crisis: Corruption." Brookings Institution, July 22, 2020. https://www.brookings .edu/research/addressing-the-other-covid-crisis-corruption/.

Phillips, Amber. 2020. "'Totally Unprecedented in Living Memory': Congress's Bipartisanship on Coronavirus Underscores What a Crisis This Is." *Washington Post,* March 26, 2020. https://www.washingtonpost.com /politics/2020/03/26/totally-unprecedented-living-memory-congresss -bipartisanship-coronavirus-underscores-what-crisis-this-is/.

Wilkie, Christina, and Amanda Macias. 2020. "Trump Removes Inspector General Overseeing $2 Trillion Coronavirus Relief Package Days after He Was Appointed." CNBC, April 7, 2020. https://www.cnbc.com/2020/04/07/coronavirus-relief-trump-removes-inspector-general-overseeing-2-trillion-package.html.

Wisconsin Holds Its Primary Election (April 7, 2020)

On March 25, 2020, Wisconsin governor Tony Evers followed the lead of other governors and issued a stay-at-home order to combat the spread of the novel coronavirus. Less than two weeks later, the swing state was scheduled to hold its primary election. Wisconsin voters would have the opportunity to express their preference among presidential hopefuls, select candidates for eight congressional districts and various state and local offices, and elect a justice to the state supreme court.

While the public health emergency prompted more than a dozen other states to cancel or postpone their primaries, Wisconsin's Democratic governor and Republican-controlled legislature engaged in heated political and legal battles to determine whether and how to conduct the election safely in the midst of a pandemic. Although the Wisconsin primary ultimately took place on April 7 despite the lockdown, critics noted that it forced residents "to make a terrible choice between shielding themselves against COVID-19 and exercising their fundamental right to vote" (Root 2020). Political analysts looked to the chaotic Wisconsin primary experience for lessons in how to adjust state election systems to reduce the risks for voters and poll workers in the November general election.

Partisan Battles Surround Election

On March 25, when confirmed COVID-19 cases in Wisconsin exceeded 450, Evers imposed a series of "safer at home" restrictions on state residents. The order required people to stay at home except for brief trips to acquire necessities such as food or medicine, to access health care services, or to exercise outdoors. It recommended that people avoid socializing with people other than members of their immediate households and maintain at least 6 feet of distance between themselves and others in public spaces. The governor called on residents "to remember our Wisconsin values of kindness, compassion, empathy, and respect" and "to do your part to keep our friends and our family and, frankly, most importantly our health care workers in communities, safe" (White 2020). The order remained in effect through April 24 and included penalties of 30 days in jail or a $250 fine for noncompliance.

As soon as the restrictions took effect, Wisconsin leaders began debating how they would impact the primary election scheduled for April 7. Public health officials warned that in-person voting—which often involved waiting in line at crowded polling locations and using pens, ballots, and voting machines that had been touched by countless other people—carried a serious risk of exposing voters to the coronavirus. They recommended adapting state voting systems to allow as many voters as possible to remain at home and cast their ballots through indirect means. Wisconsin already had election laws in place to allow for early voting and no-excuse absentee voting by mail. On March 26, Evers proposed legislation to expand these options to make voting easier and safer during the pandemic. His proposal called for increasing the number of absentee ballots being printed and distributed, suspending a requirement for absentee ballots to be signed by a witness, and accepting absentee ballots postmarked—rather than received—by election day. Republicans in the state legislature rejected the plan, however, claiming that it presented too many logistical problems.

Meanwhile, an increasing number of poll workers and voters expressed concerns about the potential health risks presented by in-person voting. Around 7,000 poll workers refused to perform their duties for fear of exposure to the coronavirus, resulting in personnel shortages that limited early voting at many polling locations—especially in large cities such as Madison and Milwaukee. In addition, more than 1.2 million Wisconsin voters requested absentee ballots—five times the number who voted absentee in the 2016 presidential election—in order to exercise their franchise while complying with the stay-at-home order (Root 2020). The massive increase in absentee voting led to confusion and turmoil. Many jurisdictions experienced shortages of ballots or envelopes, and reports later revealed that thousands of voters who requested absentee ballots never received them.

Confronted with these issues, Evers and his Democratic administration expressed a desire to either postpone the primary or forego in-person voting and conduct the election exclusively by mail. The Republican-controlled legislature dismissed these suggestions, however, and insisted on holding the election as scheduled and maintaining ordinary voting procedures. Some political analysts attributed the Republican position to the widely held belief that coronavirus concerns would mainly suppress voter turnout in hard-hit urban areas that tended to lean Democratic. State Republican leaders, on the other hand, characterized Evers's efforts to postpone the election as a political calculation that would favor Democratic candidates.

On April 4, the governor called a special session of the legislature to vote on the question of distributing absentee ballots to all registered voters. Republican lawmakers responded by gaveling the session into order and then adjourning it a few seconds later without considering Evers's request. Two days later, Evers signed an executive order postponing the primary election until June 9. Wisconsin laws made it unclear whether the governor had the authority to change election dates, rules, and procedures. State lawmakers immediately challenged the order, and the Republican-majority Wisconsin Supreme Court issued a 4-2 decision striking it down and allowing the primary to proceed on April 7 as originally scheduled. In a separate emergency ruling, the U.S. Supreme Court modified an earlier U.S. District Court decision that had extended the deadline for mailing and receiving absentee ballots to April 13. Instead, the justices ruled 5-4 that Wisconsin could only count absentee ballots that were either postmarked or hand-delivered to a polling place by election day.

Voting During a Pandemic

The legal wrangling over the election date and last-minute changes to voting procedures made it difficult for the Wisconsin Elections Commission to administer a fair and orderly primary. Local officials in many jurisdictions struggled to cope with shortages of poll workers, personal protective equipment, and sanitation supplies. Evers ended up mobilizing 2,400 members of the Wisconsin National Guard to provide election support. To promote social distancing by voters, some jurisdictions closed smaller polling stations and opened new ones in larger facilities, such as empty retail stores, industrial warehouses, or high school gymnasiums. Poll workers also marked off 6-foot distances using cones, rope, or tape and limited the number of voters allowed inside at one time. Some polling locations improvised drive-through voting procedures and distributed ballots to voters who remained in their vehicles. A voter in Beloit complained about curbside polling, however, noting that "people seemed confused by the whole process, on both sides of the clipboard" (Garcia et al. 2020).

Despite the challenges involved in voting during a pandemic, Wisconsin reported 34 percent turnout for the April 7 election—the highest for a primary in 36 years. Although a record 70 percent of voters cast absentee ballots by mail, compared to 10 percent in previous elections, many people who voted in person had to wait in long lines. In the city of Milwaukee, which reduced its polling places from 180 to 5, the average wait time to vote ranged from 1.5 to 2 hours. Voters in other districts reported waiting for up to 4 hours, placing their health at risk in the process (Garcia et al. 2020). Public health experts predicted a spike in COVID-19 cases in the weeks following the primary, and state officials confirmed 71 new positive tests among people who had voted in person or worked at polling locations. Yet researchers examining the Wisconsin election came to conflicting conclusions. One study found that higher rates of COVID-19 transmission occurred in counties with large numbers of in-person voters, but another study found no correlation.

Critics claimed that Wisconsin Republicans had resisted changing the primary date in the expectation that it would suppress Democratic turnout and benefit their candidates. In the end, however, the election results did not validate this strategy. In the main contest watched by political observers, liberal challenger Jill Karofsky upset conservative incumbent Daniel Kelly to claim a seat on the Wisconsin Supreme Court. After learning of her victory, Karofsky condemned the chaotic and politically divisive election process. "Although we were successful in this race, the circumstances under which this election was conducted were simply unacceptable, and raise serious concerns for the future of our democracy," she said. "Too many were unable to have their voices heard because they didn't feel safe leaving their home or their absentee ballots weren't counted" (Levine 2020).

As the November 2020 presidential election approached, political analysts reviewed the Wisconsin primary experience to glean insights into the changes required to ensure a safe, fair, and democratic election during a public health crisis. Although the CARES Act dedicated $400 million to election preparedness, critics asserted that billions of dollars in additional funding were needed to address the problems that occurred in Wisconsin and protect the integrity of the general election. The Center for American Progress recommended that state election officials promote vote-by-mail options, permit early voting up to 14 days before election day, allow online and same-day voter registration, and eliminate voter-identification requirements. Wisconsin applied $7.2 million of its federal CARES Act funding to shore up its election systems and procedures. State and municipal authorities also worked together to develop the Wisconsin Safe Voting Plan, which funded programs aimed at recruiting and training new poll workers, providing hazard pay for poll workers, covering sanitation expenses for polling locations, sending informational mailings to voters, and creating tracking systems for absentee ballots.

Further Reading

Epstein, Reid J. 2020. "Why Wisconsin Republicans Insisted on an Election in a Pandemic." *New York Times,* April 7, 2020. https://www.nytimes.com /2020/04/07/us/politics/wisconsin-pandemic-primary-republicans.html.

Garcia, Joaquin, Zahavah Levine, Bea Phi, Peter Prindiville, Jeff Rodriguez, Lexi Rubow, and Grace Scullion. 2020. "Wisconsin's 2020 Primary in the Wake of COVID-19." Lawfare, August 10, 2020. https://www.lawfareblog .com/wisconsins-2020-primary-wake-covid-19.

Levine, Sam. 2020. "Republicans Tried to Suppress the Vote in Wisconsin. It Backfired." *Guardian,* April 14, 2020. https://www.theguardian.com/us -news/2020/apr/14/wisconsin-election-coronavirus-republicans-supreme -court.

Root, Danielle. 2020. "Wisconsin Primary Shows Why States Must Prepare Their Elections for the Coronavirus." Center for American Progress, April 27, 2020. https://www.americanprogress.org/issues/democracy/news/2020 /04/27/484013/wisconsin-primary-shows-states-must-prepare-elections -coronavirus/.

White, Laurel. 2020. "Evers Administration Issues 'Stay-at-Home' Order for Wisconsin." Wisconsin Public Radio, March 27, 2020. https://www.wpr.org /evers-administration-issues-stay-home-order-wisconsin.

Reopening the Economy Triggers a Second Wave (May–July, 2020)

The stay-at-home orders, social-distancing measures, school closures, business shutdowns, and other restrictions that most states enacted during March and April succeeded in slowing the spread of the novel coronavirus in the United States. Such hard-hit states as New York—which peaked at more than 11,500 new cases of COVID-19 on April 14—saw their daily numbers decline to manageable levels in May. Despite their effectiveness, however, the state lockdowns disrupted the daily lives of Americans, some of whom resented being forced to hunker down and shelter in place for weeks on end.

The restrictions also took a severe toll on the U.S. economy. The unemployment rate skyrocketed from an 80-year low of 3.5 percent in February to 14.7 percent in April as the economy shed more than 20 million jobs. Retail sales plummeted by 8.7 percent from February to March—the largest monthly drop ever recorded—forcing countless stores and restaurants out of business (Bauer et al. 2020). Gross domestic product (GDP) declined at an annualized rate of 32.9 percent during the second quarter of 2020, wiping out five years' worth of economic growth (Mutikani 2020). "Whatever the public health merits, we find that lockdown policies and business closures do real damage to the economy that goes beyond the actual effects predicted by infections or deaths at the county level," wrote Brookings Institution scholars Jonathan Rothwell and Christos Makridis (2020).

As the state lockdowns wore on, President Donald Trump expressed growing impatience with the restrictions and their negative impact on the economy. He pressured the states to lift the stay-at-home orders and allow people to return to work, and he publicly feuded with governors who asserted that reopening too soon posed an unacceptable public health risk. In more than 20 states, conservative and right-wing groups organized protests against the restrictions, arguing that they extended too far and infringed upon citizens' rights and liberties. Trump tweeted his support for the anti-lockdown demonstrators, urging them to "liberate" their states. "You have a lot of, unfortunately in this case, Democrat governors, I think they think it's good politics to keep it closed," Trump stated. "I think they're being forced to open, frankly. The people want to get out. You'll break the country if you don't" (Subramanian 2020).

As governors sought to balance the need to contain the coronavirus with the desire to restore normal social and economic activity, public health experts warned that reopening states too soon could launch a second wave of COVID-19 outbreaks. "In the U.S., we had two months of essentially a lockdown [of] 90 percent of the population, but during the two months we didn't get the testing structure, contact tracing, people apparatus set up," said physician Eric Topol. "So, we are really looking for trouble. What will happen is that we're going to have to shut down again" (Oppenheimer 2020). Such predictions proved true in June, when the nation experienced daily infection rates higher than during the initial wave in March and April. Although early signs had raised hopes of a quick economic recovery, the resurgence of COVID-19 cases convinced many consumers to limit their risks by staying close to home and not patronizing newly reopened businesses.

Protests Erupt over State Lockdown Orders

The statewide stay-at-home orders put in place across most of the country in late March created challenges and hardships for many Americans. Business shutdowns resulted in mass unemployment and financial insecurity. School closures and a lack of day care options forced parents to juggle the competing demands of online learning, childcare, and working from home. Families struggled to adapt to constant togetherness or made the difficult choice to avoid in-person gatherings with vulnerable members. Individuals grappled with depression and other mental health issues stemming from isolation, fear, and uncertainty.

Some people reacted to the state lockdown orders with frustration, anger, and resentment. Critics pointed out that most COVID-19 cases tended to be centered in densely populated urban areas, so they questioned whether it made sense to impose the same restrictions on sparsely populated rural regions. They also noted that certain population groups— including older Americans and those with certain preexisting medical conditions—appeared to face a much greater risk of death from COVID-19 than young, healthy Americans. Some suggested limiting stay-at-home orders to vulnerable groups while allowing low-risk populations to resume their normal activities. Other opponents of state lockdowns expressed doubts about the severity of the coronavirus and argued that authorities should allow it to spread among healthier Americans to establish herd immunity. Some described the stringent measures as exceedingly harmful to the nation's economic health, citing the adage that the cure should not be worse than the disease. Finally, some opponents objected to government-imposed restrictions as unconstitutional infringements on the American people's fundamental rights and freedoms.

Many critics shared their grievances on social media, and conservative and right-wing groups organized public anti-lockdown demonstrations in nearly two dozen states. The first such protest, dubbed Operation Gridlock, took place on April 15 in Lansing, Michigan. An estimated 3,000 people turned out to express their displeasure with the restrictions imposed by Governor Gretchen Whitmer (D) in her effort to slow the spread of the coronavirus. Although most people remained in their vehicles and blocked the streets surrounding the state capitol building, a few hundred protesters gathered on the lawn and sidewalk. Many ignored the governor's recommendations to wear protective face masks and observe social distancing. "I don't think that we need the Constitution suspended in order to be safe," said one protester. "It's a personal responsibility regardless. My point is that we don't need it imposed upon us. The American people are smart enough to be able to make these decisions themselves" (Hutchinson 2020).

Over the next few weeks, similar demonstrations took place in other hard-hit states led by Democratic governors. In Washington, for instance, protesters expressed their objections to the restrictions imposed by Governor Jay Inslee. Trump expressed support for the anti-lockdown protesters. "These people love our country, they want to get back to work," he stated. "Their life was taken away from them." Inslee responded by accusing the president of "fomenting domestic rebellion" against policies recommended by U.S. public health officials (BBC News 2020). Supporters of the aggressive pandemic response mounted by state governors derided the anti-lockdown protests as anti-science, a threat to public health, and disrespectful to the frontline workers putting themselves at risk to help others during the crisis. "These protests here are so discouraging," said Minnesota intensive care nurse Mary Turner. "With no one doing social distancing or wearing masks, and they all say they are outraged. I don't know if this is a problem anywhere else in the world" (Maqbool 2020).

Polls showed that the protests represented a minority viewpoint in the United States. A Pew Research Center survey found that only one-third of Americans believed that the stay-at-home orders should be lifted more quickly, while two-thirds worried that the restrictions would be relaxed before the virus had abated (BBC News 2020). Research also suggested that much of the opposition to state lockdowns was rooted in political beliefs or ideology. Media coverage of the anti-lockdown demonstrations noted that they often resembled Trump campaign rallies, with protesters carrying pro-Trump flags and banners and wearing "Make America Great Again" shirts and hats. Gun rights activists and self-identified militia members played a prominent role in many of the demonstrations as well. On April 30, for instance, a group of gun owners carried assault weapons into the Michigan capitol and interrupted a session of the state legislature.

Some political analysts noted that the anti-lockdown protests coincided with the release of demographic data showing that people of color accounted for a disproportionate number of COVID-related deaths in the United States. Studies revealed that nearly 60 percent of all coronavirus deaths nationwide occurred in counties with majority black populations. Researchers cited racial health disparities, limited access to quality medical care, and higher transmission risk in densely populated urban areas as factors in the increased morbidity rates. They also noted that black and Latino Americans were overrepresented in essential jobs—in grocery stores, nursing homes, farms, and factories—with a high risk of exposure to the coronavirus and little opportunity to work remotely. According to some critics, the fact that COVID-19 disproportionately impacted communities of color provided political cover for Trump and his allies in the conservative media to advocate reopening the economy and putting people back to work. "That more and more Americans were dying was less important than who was dying," Adam Serwer (2020) wrote in the *Atlantic*. "Public-health restrictions designed to contain the outbreak were deemed absurd. . . . To restrict the freedom of white Americans, just because nonwhite Americans are dying, is an egregious violation of the racial contract."

Reopened States See Coronavirus Surge

On April 16, Trump's White House Coronavirus Task Force released guidelines for easing restrictions and reopening the U.S. economy. The guidelines recommended that states reopen in three phases as they attained target numbers for COVID-19 cases. Some critics pointed out that the guidelines assumed states would see a steady reduction in cases and offered little advice for responding to new outbreaks. "It was all predicated on reduction, open, reduction, open more, reduction, open," said Francis X. Suarez, the Republican mayor of Miami, Florida. "There was never what happens if there is an increase after you reopen?" (Shear et al. 2020). Upon reviewing the federal guidelines, some public health experts warned that they pushed states to reopen too quickly—before comprehensive testing and contact tracing protocols were put in place—and increased the risk for uncontrolled spread of the coronavirus. Some governors refused to follow the Trump administration's recommendations and instead established their own benchmarks for reopening safely.

But in many states—especially in the South—Republican governors who had resisted imposing stay-at-home orders began relaxing or eliminating restrictions in late April and early May. South Carolina allowed retail businesses to reopen on April 20, making it the first state to lift shutdown measures. Georgia followed suit four days later, and Texas, Florida, and Arizona began reopening in early May. Texas Governor Greg Abbott allowed retail stores, restaurants, movie theaters, and malls to reopen on May 1 with reduced capacity and special rules in place. He expanded the reopening plan to include bars on May 18, just in time for Memorial Day weekend. Over the next two weeks, young Texans took advantage of their newfound freedom by packing into popular nightclubs in defiance of social-distancing guidelines. In Arizona, where Governor Doug Ducey rescinded his stay-at-home order and allowed restaurants to reopen on May 8, many establishments saw long lines of patrons congregating without protective face masks.

Most states that reopened quickly experienced an immediate increase in consumer spending and decrease in unemployment. However, they also began seeing a rise in coronavirus cases in late May and June. South Carolina reported an increase of nearly 1,000 percent in daily COVID-19 cases, from an average of 143 per day at reopening to an average of 1,570 per day by late June. Likewise, Florida reported an increase in daily cases of nearly 1,400 percent, and Arizona experienced an increase of more than 850 percent (Gamio 2020). Nationwide, the number of confirmed cases surged above 75,000 per day—twice as high as the peak daily rates in mid-April—prompting some public health officials to declare a second wave underway. Critics noted that the resurgence of the coronavirus largely centered in the states that reopened early, while those that adopted a slower, more cautious approach appeared to fare better. In New York—which served as the original epicenter of the pandemic in the United States—Governor Andrew Cuomo waited until late May to take the first tentative steps toward reopening. Daily COVID-19 case rates declined by more than 50 percent afterward, and only about 1 percent of coronavirus tests conducted in New York returned positive results, compared to the national average of 9 percent (Gamio 2020).

Trump attributed the spike in COVID-19 cases to increased testing. He claimed that the apparent growth in numbers occurred because more cases were being diagnosed rather than because the coronavirus was spreading. "We're going to have more cases because we do more testing. Otherwise, you don't know if you have a case," he stated. "So, in a way, by doing all of this testing, we make ourselves look bad" (Trump 2020). Public health experts rejected this explanation, however. Even though the United States tripled its testing capacity between April and June, the increase in cases outpaced the increase in testing in half of all states (Gamio 2020).

Public health officials initially blamed the surge on the resumption of social activities in states that reopened quickly. They noted that the majority of second-wave cases seemed to be concentrated among younger adults who took fewer precautions and flocked to crowded bars, restaurants, and house parties as soon as the restrictions were lifted. In late June, however, the U.S. Centers for Disease Control and Prevention (CDC) acknowledged that it had severely underestimated the number of coronavirus cases circulating in the spring. "The virus was in fact spreading with invisible ferocity during the weeks in May when states were opening up with Mr. Trump's encouragement and many were all but declaring victory," according to an analysis in the *New York Times* (Shear et al. 2020).

Facing a resurgence of COVID-19 cases that threatened to overwhelm hospitals, more than one-third of states had to pause their reopening plans or reinstate some restrictions. Texas shut down its bars, for instance, and Florida prohibited its bars from serving alcohol. Some states that successfully contained their outbreaks instituted travel restrictions or quarantine orders targeting the new coronavirus hot spots. West Virginia Jim Justice (R) urged residents of his state to avoid vacationing in South Carolina, while the governors of New York, New Jersey, and Connecticut issued a joint travel advisory asking residents to self-quarantine for two weeks after visiting certain hard-hit states in the South.

States with rising COVID-19 cases saw economic activity slow down, based on such indicators as consumer spending, restaurant patronage, and employment levels. Even in states that did not reverse their decisions to reopen, the resurgence of the virus made many people reluctant to resume their old patterns of socializing, spending, and traveling. According to a Deutsche Bank analysis, "The lesson is that behavioral changes in response to COVID trends can hinder the economic recovery even if states do not reimpose containment measures" (Picchi 2020). Some analysts argued that unsuccessful reopening attempts lowered consumer confidence and convinced more Americans to stay home until a vaccine became available. "Even though it won't be everyone at once, people might just throw up their hands, say 'you know what, it is not worth it,'" said Raphael Bostic, president of the Federal Reserve Bank of Atlanta. "'I will just do my take-out. I will do Netflix instead of going to the movies'" (Schneider 2020). The second wave of COVID-19 thus threatened to undermine the national economic recovery that Trump had hoped to achieve by reopening the states.

Even as some states managed to contain the second wave of outbreaks, some observers predicted that the country would experience another resurgence in the fall as schools reopened and colder weather forced people indoors. "The surge of COVID-19 cases and deaths in America over the summer resulted from a toxic mix of factors: states reopening, lockdown fatigue, and a season typically filled with vacations and holidays," according to German Lopez (2020) of Vox. "People gathered and celebrated indoors—at bars, restaurants, and friends' and family's homes. Millions of people got sick, and tens of thousands died. This fall, experts worry it will all happen again: States are rolling back restrictions, people are eager to get back to normal, and Thanksgiving and Christmas are coming up. America may be on the verge of repeating the same mistakes, which would risk yet another surge in the COVID-19 epidemic."

Further Reading

Bauer, Lauren, Kristen E. Broady, Wendy Edelberg, and Jimmy O'Donnell. 2020. "Ten Facts about COVID-19 and the U.S. Economy." Brookings Institution, September 17, 2020. https://www.brookings.edu/research/ten-facts -about-covid-19-and-the-u-s-economy/.

BBC News. 2020. "Coronavirus Lockdown Protests: What's Behind the U.S. Protests?" BBC, April 21, 2020. https://www.bbc.com/news/world-us-canada -52359100.

Gamio, Lazaro. 2020. "How Coronavirus Cases Have Risen since States Reopened." *New York Times*, July 9, 2020. https://www.nytimes.com /interactive/2020/07/09/us/coronavirus-cases-reopening-trends.html.

Hutchinson, Bill. 2020. "'Operation Gridlock': Convoy in Michigan's Capital Protests Stay-at-Home Orders." ABC News, April 1, 2020. https://abcnews.go

.com/US/convoy-protesting-stay-home-orders-targets-michigans-capital /story?id=70138816.

Lopez, German. 2020. "Experts Say COVID-19 Cases Are Likely about to Surge." Vox, October 5, 2020. https://www.vox.com/future-perfect/2020/9/28 /21451436/covid-19-coronavirus-pandemic-fall-winter-third-wave.

Maqbool, Aleem. 2020. "Coronavirus: The U.S. Resistance to a Continued Lockdown." BBC News, April 27, 2020. https://www.bbc.com/news/world-us -canada-52417610.

Mutikani, Lucia. 2020. "What to Know about the Report on America's COVID-Hit GDP." World Economic Forum, July 31, 2020. https://www.weforum .org/agenda/2020/07/covid-19-coronavirus-usa-united-states-econamy -gdp-decline/.

Oppenheimer, Andres. 2020. "The Way Trump Reopened Economy Will Likely Spur a Second Wave of COVID-19." *Miami Herald,* June 6, 2020. https:// www.miamiherald.com/news/local/news-columns-blogs/andres -oppenheimer/article243331476.html#storylink=cpy.

Picchi, Aimee. 2020. "Coronavirus Surge in States That Rushed to Reopen Is Hurting Economic Growth." CBS News, June 29, 2020. https://www.cbsnews .com/news/coronavirus-states-rushed-reopen-hurting-economic-growth/.

Rothwell, Jonathan, and Christos Makridis. 2020. "Politics Is Wrecking America's Pandemic Response." Brookings Institution, September 17, 2020. https://www.brookings.edu/blog/up-front/2020/09/17/politics-is -wrecking-americas-pandemic-response/.

Schneider, Howard. 2020. "A Quick Reopening, a Surge in Infections, and a U.S. Recovery at Risk." Reuters, June 26, 2020. https://www.reuters.com/article /us-usa-economy-recovery-analysis/a-quick-reopening-a-surge-in -infections-and-a-u-s-recovery-at-risk-idUSKBN23X2CF.

Serwer, Adam. 2020. "The Coronavirus Was an Emergency until Trump Found Out Who Was Dying." *Atlantic,* May 8, 2020. https://www.theatlantic .com/ideas/archive/2020/05/americas-racial-contract-showing/611389/.

Shear, Michael D., Noah Weiland, Eric Lipton, Maggie Haberman, and David E. Sanger. 2020. "Inside Trump's Failure: The Rush to Abandon Leadership Role on the Virus." *New York Times,* July 19, 2020. https://www.nytimes .com/2020/07/18/us/politics/trump-coronavirus-response-failure -leadership.html.

Subramanian, Courtney. 2020. "Trump Accuses Democratic Governors of Keeping Lockdowns Because of 'Politics' as He Visits Michigan." *USA Today,* May 21, 2020. https://www.usatoday.com/story/news/politics/2020/05/21 /coronavirus-trump-blasts-democrats-over-lockdowns-michigan-visit /5235638002/.

Trump, Donald. 2020. "Remarks by President Trump and Vice President Pence at a Meeting with Governor Reynolds of Iowa." The White House, May 6, 2020. https://www.whitehouse.gov/briefings-statements/remarks-president -trump-vice-president-pence-meeting-governor-reynolds-iowa/.

CHAPTER THREE

Impacts of the COVID-19 Pandemic

This chapter examines the impact of the COVID-19 pandemic on American society. It reviews the fundamental changes to home and family life precipitated by stay-at-home orders, online learning, and an unprecedented atmosphere of fear, uncertainty, and loss. It also explores the effects of prolonged school closures on the education and development of American children and college students. Finally, the chapter analyzes how politics and partisanship shaped the government's response to the pandemic as well as citizens' compliance with mask wearing, social distancing, and other mitigation measures.

Home and Family Life

Beginning in March 2020, state and local officials imposed a series of coronavirus lockdown orders that eventually affected more than three-quarters of the U.S. population, or around 250 million Americans. Most of these measures closed schools and nonessential businesses, canceled sporting and cultural events, prohibited residents from gathering in groups, and urged people to remain at home except to purchase food, access medical care, or exercise outdoors. Although the widespread stay-at-home orders proved effective in "flattening the curve," or lowering daily COVID-19 case counts to levels that did not overwhelm hospital capacity, they also disrupted the daily lives of individuals and families and precipitated a severe economic downturn. Growing public frustration with the lockdown orders, combined with political pressure to reopen the economy, led to a gradual easing of restrictions in most parts of the country in May and June. Even as COVID-19 cases surged to new heights in the summer and fall, however, few Americans seemed willing to repeat the lockdown experience. "America does not have the willpower or the leadership to withstand another shutdown or more economic devastation," said public health expert Daniel B. Fagbuyi (Curley 2020).

Lockdowns Disrupt Americans' Daily Lives

The stay-at-home orders that affected most of the country in the early spring of 2020 created challenges and hardships for millions of Americans. In a Pew Research Center poll released on March 30, 90 percent of respondents said that their life had changed at least somewhat due to the measures implemented to curb the spread of the coronavirus (Parker 2020). Many people went into virtual quarantine with their partners or immediate family members, only leaving home on brief errands to pick up groceries or walk the dog. For members of shared households, the lockdowns brought them into constant contact without the relief usually provided by outside activities and separate support networks. For people who lived alone, on the other hand, staying at home meant isolation from friends, family, and the wider community. "Old activities like socializing, going to the gym, eating out, are no longer available options to us," noted clinical psychologist Sharmeen Shroff (Liu 2020).

To fill the hours, days, and weeks of "nesting" at home, Americans turned to binge-watching television programs, movies, and live-streamed online content. Musicians, comedians, and other entertainers filmed performances in their living rooms and shared the footage with fans. Board games, puzzles, books, and hobby and craft supplies sold out online as millions of people sought comfort and camaraderie in traditional forms of entertainment from less stressful times. Many people tackled home improvement projects or took up gardening or cooking. Parks, trails, and beaches emerged as popular venues for socially-distanced exercise with the cancelation of sports leagues and the closure of gyms and pools. Animal adoptions soared at shelters across the country as lonely people sought safe companionship in pets. Some people responded to the fear and uncertainty by turning to religion. According to the Pew survey, 55 percent of respondents said they prayed for an end to pandemic—including 24 percent who did not belong to any organized religion—although 59 percent of regular churchgoers said they stopped attending religious services due to coronavirus concerns (Parker 2020).

With 42 percent of Americans reporting health concerns about going to the grocery store (Parker 2020), online shopping, grocery delivery services, and curbside pickup options exploded in popularity. People who did their own grocery shopping tended to make less frequent trips, stay closer to home, and purchase more non-perishable food items and household cleaning supplies. As lockdowns made the severity of the public health crisis clear, many people panicked and began hoarding toilet paper, hand sanitizer, disinfectant wipes, protective face masks, and other supplies. Shortages of these materials left store shelves empty and led to long delivery delays on Amazon and other e-commerce sites. Even as some states began to relax restrictions, 77 percent of Americans said they felt uncomfortable about dining in a restaurant (Parker 2020). Instead, people increasingly cooked meals at home or ordered carryout or delivery.

The Pew survey found that 40 percent of all working-age adults began working remotely from home during the lockdowns, with the proportion increasing to 73 percent for people with advanced degrees (Parker 2020). As a result, usage of videoconferencing technology grew by a factor of 20 within three months (Kohli et al. 2020). At the same time, however, the business closures and resulting economic downturn triggered huge job losses, with more than 14 million Americans filing for unemployment compensation during the early months of the pandemic. The job losses were more pronounced among low-income workers, nearly half of whom reported having trouble paying their bills after the coronavirus lockdowns started (Parker, Minkin, and Bennett 2020). People classified as essential workers—which encompassed such sectors as food and agriculture, transportation, manufacturing, utilities, and government services as well as health care—continued to report to work despite the risk of exposure to the coronavirus.

With schools closed and most day care facilities reserved for the children of essential workers, many working parents struggled to balance the demands of their jobs with the needs of their children. Some families reported positive outcomes from forced togetherness, with parents devising more equitable divisions of work, housework, and childcare and children thriving under regular routines and increased parental attention. Other families experienced increased levels of tension and conflict. "The anxiety and uncertainty of the current situation add further stress to the changed dynamics families are having to cope with," said New York University psychiatrist Andrew E. Roffman (NYU Langone 2020). Some family conflicts arose out of differing opinions about how carefully to observe stay-at-home orders and social-distancing measures. "Now, mundane discussions between couples like 'should we send our child to this play date' have become matters of life and death," Shroff explained, "[w]hich will inevitably put families under strain and relationships to the test" (Liu 2020).

For some couples, constant togetherness under lockdown orders damaged or exposed existing rifts in their relationships. One study found that the U.S. divorce rate for March–June 2020 increased by 34 percent over the same period a year earlier (Rosner 2020). Mandatory stay-at-home orders also posed risks for people in unsafe living conditions or abusive relationships by making it impossible for them to avoid or escape danger. The additional stress caused by social isolation, job loss, financial insecurity, and coronavirus concerns contributed to a significant increase in the incidence and severity of domestic violence. "The person choosing to use violence—the perpetrator—employs violence as a tool to establish and maintain power and control over their partner," said Barbara Paradiso, director of the Center on Domestic Violence at the University of Colorado. "That need for power is, in part, a reflection of the lack of power they feel over their environment. COVID has brought with it just about every uncertainty any of us can imagine: Will we lose our jobs? Be furloughed? When will be allowed to go back to work or school? Can I make my rent payment? And on and on. That lack of control each of us are feeling is likely to be amplified for the abuser, and so they amplify their violence" (Mozes 2020).

The coronavirus and efforts to contain it also impacted friendships and social rituals. Staying at home during the pandemic inspired some people to reestablish lost connections with distant friends and relatives through social media, online videoconferencing, or simple telephone calls. Others took the opportunity to reevaluate their relationships and shift their focus from cultivating a wide circle to nurturing a few important friendships. In some cases, negotiations and disagreements over COVID-19 precautions revealed fundamental differences in friends' personalities and outlooks. While one friend might suggest patronizing a favorite bar or restaurant as soon as it reopened, for instance, another might insist on meeting outdoors, remaining 6 feet apart, and wearing masks. "We're faced with a moment with our friends in which we're having to navigate consent like people do with sexual relationships," said science journalist Lydia Denworth (Ellison 2020). Even after restrictions were lifted, many people canceled, postponed, or significantly altered plans for weddings, graduations, vacations, and other social events. Others asserted their right to associate freely despite the risks it might pose to the community.

The atmosphere of fear and uncertainty—combined with feelings of loneliness, boredom, hardship, and loss—caused psychological distress for many people during the pandemic and associated shutdowns. In a series of surveys by the Kaiser Family Foundation, the percentage of American adults reporting negative impacts on their mental health increased from 32 percent in March to 53 percent in July. More than one-third of respondents experienced difficulty sleeping due to stress, while 12 percent experienced a worsening of chronic health conditions (Chidambaram 2020). Many people turned to alcohol to help relieve feelings of anxiety and depression brought on by coronavirus lockdowns. Alcohol sales increased by 26 percent nationwide between March and June, and surveys showed that many Americans—especially women—increased both the frequency and amount of their alcohol consumption. Some experts expressed concerns about a spate of substance abuse disorders arising from the pandemic. "I think that the shelter-in-place aspect has had devastating and long-term effects—many that we haven't seen the full results from yet," said Kurtis Taylor of the Alcohol/Drug Council of North Carolina. "People are developing issues that will not be easily shaken" (Lukpat 2020).

United States Reluctant to Reinstate Lockdowns

By some estimates, the stay-at-home orders enacted in the spring of 2020 prevented up to 60 million Americans from contracting COVID-19 (Curley 2020). Nevertheless, the toll that the lockdowns exacted on individuals, families, and the U.S. economy largely eliminated the political will to impose further restrictions to contain future COVID-19 outbreaks. "There does not seem to be any appetite from governors, the [President Donald Trump] administration, or Congress to encourage a second wave of stay-at-home orders if we can continue to take alternate measures to curb the spread, such as encouraging mask wearing, social distancing, and other public health actions," said health care policy adviser Heather Meade (Curley 2020).

Against the advice of public health experts, Trump began pressuring states to lift restrictions in April in the interest of reopening businesses and restoring U.S. economic health. Trump supporters played a prominent role in organizing anti-lockdown protests in many states—especially those led by Democratic governors—claiming that the restrictions violated their constitutional rights and personal liberties and caused unnecessary harm to businesses and the economy. As daily COVID-19 case counts declined in May, most states established reopening plans that gradually phased out restrictions. Although millions of Americans continued taking such precautions as wearing masks and social distancing, many others viewed the crisis as over and sought to resume their normal lives. Younger adults, in particular, demonstrated an eagerness to patronize crowded bars and nightclubs as soon as they reopened.

By mid-June, the number of U.S. COVID-19 cases surged above 75,000 per day—twice as many as during the previous peak in mid-April—prompting some public health officials to declare a second wave of infections underway. Critics noted that the resurgence of the coronavirus largely centered in the states that reopened early, while those that adopted a slower, more cautious approach appeared to fare better. On the other hand, the earlier-reopening states experienced quicker economic recoveries, boasting lower unemployment rates and higher consumer spending. Few states imposed strict new measures to contain the outbreaks, partly due to a lack of public support for another round of lockdowns. "The appetite for shutting down the entire country is simply not there," said epidemiologist Farley Cleghorn (Curley 2020).

Further Reading

Chidambaram, Priya. 2020. "The Implications of COVID-19 for Mental Health and Substance Use." Kaiser Family Foundation, August 21, 2020. https://www.kff.org/coronavirus-covid-19/issue-brief/the-implications-of-covid-19-for-mental-health-and-substance-use/.

Curley, Christopher. 2020. "It's Unlikely the U.S. Will Have Another COVID-19 Lockdown No Matter How High the Numbers Get." Healthline, September 30, 2020. https://www.healthline.com/health-news/its-unlikely-the-us-will-have-another-covid-19-lockdown-no-matter-how-high-the-numbers-get.

Ellison, Katherine. 2020. "Stress from the Pandemic Can Destroy Relationships with Friends—Even Families." *Washington Post,* August 7, 2020. https://www.washingtonpost.com/health/stress-from-the-pandemic-can-destroy-relationships-with-friends—even-families/2020/08/07/d95216f4-d665-11ea-aff6-220dd3a14741_story.html.

Kohli, Sajal, Björn Timelin, Victor Fabius, and Sofia Moulvad Veran. 2020. "How COVID-19 Is Changing Consumer Behavior—Now and Forever." McKinsey and Company, July 30, 2020. https://www.mckinsey.com/~/media/mckinsey/industries/retail/our%20insights/how%20covid%2019%20is%20changing%20consumer%20behavior%20now%20and%20forever/how-covid-19-is-changing-consumer-behaviornow-and-forever.pdf.

Liu, Yi-Ling. 2020. "Is COVID-19 Changing Our Relationships?" BBC Future, June 4, 2020. https://www.bbc.com/future/article/20200601-how-is-covid-19-is-affecting-relationships.

Lukpat, Alyssa. 2020. "Alcohol during the Pandemic: Study Breaks Down Who's Drinking More, and How Much." *Seattle Times,* July 20, 2020. https://www.seattletimes.com/nation-world/alcohol-during-the-pandemic-study-breaks-down-whos-drinking-more-and-how-much/.

Mozes, Alan. 2020. "Study Finds Rise in Domestic Violence during COVID." WebMD, August 18, 2020. https://www.webmd.com/lung/news/20200818

/radiology-study-suggests-horrifying-rise-in-domestic-violence-during
-pandemic#1.

NYU Langone. 2020. "A Work in Progress: Family Resilience and COVID-19."
https://nyulangone.org/news/work-progress-family-resilience-covid-19.

Parker, Kim. 2020. "Most Americans Say Coronavirus Outbreak Has Impacted
Their Lives." Pew Research Center, March 30, 2020. https://www.pew
socialtrends.org/2020/03/30/most-americans-say-coronavirus-outbreak
-has-impacted-their-lives/.

Parker, Kim, Rachel Minkin, and Jesse Bennett. 2020. "Economic Fallout from
COVID-19 Continues to Hit Lower-Income Americans the Hardest." Pew
Research Center, September 24, 2020. https://www.pewsocialtrends.org
/2020/09/24/economic-fallout-from-covid-19-continues-to-hit-lower
-income-americans-the-hardest/.

Rosner, Elizabeth. 2020. "U.S. Divorce Rates Skyrocket amid COVID-19 Pandemic." *New York Post,* September 1, 2020. https://nypost.com/2020/09
/01/divorce-rates-skyrocket-in-u-s-amid-covid-19/.

Education

When state governors shut down businesses and ordered residents to
stay at home in an effort to contain the coronavirus pandemic, they also
closed schools. Although school-aged children and young adults appeared
less likely to develop severe cases of COVID-19 than older people, public
health experts warned that allowing large numbers of students to congregate in close proximity increased the risk of spreading the virus within
schools and then on to family members and the wider community. As a
result, most U.S. public and private K–12 schools (those offering instruction to children from kindergarten through twelfth grade) temporarily
suspended in-person instruction in mid-March 2020. By early May, 48
states had closed their schools through the remainder of the academic
year ("The Coronavirus Spring" 2020). The unprecedented school closures disrupted learning and development for more than 50 million students nationwide and presented many challenges for their families.

Beginning with the University of Washington on March 6, more than
1,100 institutions of higher learning in all 50 states canceled in-person
classes and shut down on-campus housing. Some 14 million college students suddenly found themselves scrambling to pack their belongings,
arrange transportation, and return home or find other places to stay.
Although most institutions quickly transitioned to online classes, many
students felt that the remote learning approach did not justify the high
tuition rates they paid for a residential college experience. Declining
enrollment triggered by the pandemic created major financial challenges

for universities that threatened to disrupt the higher education system in the United States.

Even as COVID-19 cases continued to surge in the summer of 2020, President Donald Trump declared his intention for K–12 schools and colleges and universities to reopen in time for the fall semester. He asserted that sending students back to school was essential to getting people back to work and launching the nation's economic recovery. Trump encountered resistance from governors, teachers' unions, and parents who expressed concern that reopening schools without adequate precautions could jeopardize public health. Schools adopted a variety of strategies for limiting the risks associated with reopening, such as requiring students and staff members to wear masks, arranging classrooms to promote social distancing, staggering schedules to reduce the number of students in buildings, and utilizing outdoor spaces for group activities.

K–12 School Closures Disrupt Learning

Local K–12 school districts began closing in response to coronavirus outbreaks in late February. By the time the World Health Organization (WHO) declared COVID-19 a pandemic on March 11, more than one million American students had already been affected. On March 12, Ohio became the first state to temporarily shut down all of its K–12 schools. "We have a responsibility to save lives," Governor Mike DeWine (R) said in announcing the decision. "We could have waited to close schools, but based on advice from health experts, this is the time to do it" ("The Coronavirus Spring" 2020). Fifteen more states followed suit the next day, and on March 17 Kansas became the first state to close its schools through the end of the academic year.

All across the country, K–12 schools struggled to transition to distance learning. Many students lacked access to suitable technology or a reliable internet connection, and many school districts lacked the funding and resources to provide computers, tablets, and Wi-Fi equipment. Many educators had trouble adapting lesson plans, assignments, and assessments to an online format. Especially in lower elementary grades, teachers relied on personalized instruction and hands-on activities to engage students. The inability to apply such techniques in virtual classroom settings made it difficult for some students to pay attention and remain motivated. Many students missed the social interaction they received at school, which also contributed to their growth and development. High school students faced the postponement or cancellation of major events and educational milestones, such as sports championships, theatrical performances, spring trips, proms, and graduation ceremonies. Disappointment over the loss of these traditional rites of passage, combined with isolation and uncertainty during school closures and stay-at-home orders, posed a threat to teens' mental health.

As K–12 schools worked to make curricula available online, they encountered particular challenges in accommodating the special needs of students with disabilities. Federal law required school districts to provide these students with services outlined in their individualized education plans (IEP), which might include one-on-one support from aides, tutors, paraprofessionals, speech therapists, or physical therapists. Although some schools attempted to continue such services remotely, many lacked the personnel and resources to do so during the pandemic. A May 2020 survey by the disability organization ParentsTogether found that only 20 percent of families felt their children received the special education services to which they were entitled, while 40 percent reported that they received no services at all (North 2020). Yet reopening schools and returning to in-person classes carried risks for students with disabilities as well, since many had underlying medical conditions that made them more vulnerable to complications from COVID-19.

School closings presented many challenges for families, as children adapted to online learning and parents adjusted to having children at home during the day. Parents allowed to work from home struggled to perform their jobs while also caring for infants, entertaining small children, or overseeing the virtual schoolwork of older children and teens. Many working parents sacrificed sleep in order to meet the needs of their children during the daytime hours and fulfill the demands of their employers at night. Other parents lost or were forced to quit their jobs due to a lack of childcare options, causing their families to experience the additional stress of financial hardship. Parents who worked in essential jobs—whether at hospitals, pharmacies, grocery stores, farms, factories, or utility companies—had to arrange emergency childcare for school-age children to be able to perform their critical functions. Many states allowed nursery schools, day care facilities, churches and charitable organizations, and public recreation departments to continue to provide care for the children of essential workers. Some states offered subsidized childcare for parents directly involved in the coronavirus response.

School closures had a disproportionate impact on students from underprivileged backgrounds. These students often lacked access to digital learning resources and relied on personal interaction with teachers to help them focus and stay motivated. Since many at-risk students came from households where adult family members had limited education, they were less likely to have access to educational opportunities outside of school. Children from low-income families thus faced a greater risk of falling behind academically and dropping out of school as a result of protracted school closures. In addition, more than 30 million disadvantaged children in the United States receive free or reduced cost food at school through the National School Lunch Program. This program provides food-insecure children with healthy meals that can supply up to half of their daily caloric intake (CDC 2020). Although many school districts established programs to make food available to students during the pandemic, extended school closures posed a threat to the nutritional health and well-being of low-income students.

In addition to the short-term challenges to students and families, K–12 school closures also affected long-term learning outcomes, skill development, and economic productivity. Studies examining children's academic retention over summer vacation showed that third-graders lost around one-fourth of the reading and math skills they gained during the school year, on average, while seventh-graders lost up to half of their school-year gains (CDC 2020). Experts predicted that pandemic-related school closures—which extended for at least ten weeks in most of the country—would magnify this effect. One study estimated that the loss of one-third of a year of schooling for the nation's K–12 students in 2020 would result in a cumulative loss of long-term skills and productivity that would reduce gross domestic product (GDP) by 1.5 percent for the remainder of the century, precipitating a total economic loss of $15 trillion (Schleicher 2020). Researchers predicted that other countries would experience similar economic effects, since school closures affected 99 percent of students worldwide—or around 1.7 billion learners—in April 2020.

School Districts Wrestle with Reopening

Throughout the spring and summer of 2020, administrators of K–12 school districts debated about reopening, established guidelines and timetables, and developed strategies to mitigate the risk of COVID-19 outbreaks. Public health experts recommended placing school reopening within the context of a larger plan, implemented at the state or national level, for gradually easing other restrictions. "Everything that reopens will add to the infection rate," Vox writer German Lopez (2020) explained. "Some places may have tiny, even negligible effects, such as parks. Some are bigger threats, like bars and indoor dining. And some may carry potentially high risk but still seem worth it to the community for their social benefits, like schools. The goal, then, is to balance out a reopening—doing it slowly,

making it possible to see the effects of each extra step—to make sure outbreaks don't get out of control."

The U.S. Centers for Disease Control and Prevention (CDC) released a
School Decision Tree to help administrators weigh factors to consider in
reopening, such as the number and trajectory of COVID-19 cases in the
surrounding community. In late June, the CDC issued recommendations
for reopening safely that called for modifying classrooms to increase
space or insert barriers between seats, closing communal spaces, staggering schedules, and requiring face coverings. Trump expressed his displeasure with the guidelines on Twitter, calling them "tough," "expensive,"
and "impractical" (Klein and Liptak 2020). CDC director Robert Redfield
responded by emphasizing the importance of returning children to school
and announcing that the agency planned to revise and reissue its recommendations. "Remember it's guidance, it's not requirements, and its purpose is to facilitate the reopening and keeping open the schools in this
country," he stated (Klein and Liptak 2020). The revised CDC guidelines
emphasized the low risk the coronavirus posed to school-age children—
with only 64 deaths among Americans under age 18 attributed to COVID-
19 through mid-July—and the many benefits in-person school attendance
provided for children's educational, social, emotional, behavioral, and
physical health (CDC 2020).

Even as COVID-19 case counts reached record levels nationwide in
July, Trump pressured governors to reopen schools as usual. He claimed
that resistance to his reopening plans was politically motivated and threatened to withhold federal funding from states that did not follow his timetable. "The Dems think it would be bad for them politically if U.S. schools
open before the November Election, but is important for the children &
families," he tweeted. "May cut off funding if not open!" (Collinson 2020).
Although critics pointed out that state and local governments supplied
more than 90 percent of school funding, they acknowledged that Trump
could follow through on his threat by delaying distribution of the $13 bil-
lion in CARES Act funds dedicated to helping school districts cover costs
associated with COVID-19 preparedness.

States adopted many different approaches to reopening schools. Oregon
allowed schools to resume in-person classes when counties recorded fewer
than 10 cases per 100,000 residents for three weeks, while Arizona set a
threshold of less than 100 cases per 100,000 residents for two weeks.
Georgia reopened its schools in mid-August despite recording 189 cases
per 100,000 people the previous week (Parshley 2020). While most states
left reopening decisions to local officials, Florida was among a handful
of states that required all schools to reopen. Critics noted that Florida

experienced a 26 percent increase in COVID-19 cases among children under age 18 within the next few weeks (Schweigershausen 2020). Meanwhile, hundreds of large school districts across the country started the fall term remotely. New York delayed the start of school for several weeks and then adopted a hybrid model, in which students attended in-person classes a few days per week and took online classes on other days. Schools that reopened implemented a number of measures to reduce close contact between individuals, such as staggering arrival and dismissal times, increasing space between desks, eating lunch in classrooms rather than cafeterias, and canceling assemblies and sporting events. Other common hygiene precautions included requiring face masks, providing hand sanitizer, performing temperature checks and symptom screenings, and disinfecting classrooms regularly.

Higher Education Struggles with the Coronavirus

The coronavirus pandemic forced the temporary closure of nearly all institutions of higher learning in the United States. Many colleges and universities made the decision to close quickly, suddenly shifting their message from reassuring students that campus housing would remain open to informing students that they had to move out. At schools across the country, students who left campus for spring break were told not to return or were allowed back during brief windows to collect their belongings. Some universities kept limited housing open for international students— many of whom could not return home due to travel restrictions or visa requirements—and for students who were homeless or had no safe housing alternatives.

Liberty University, a private, evangelical Christian institution in Lynchburg, Virginia, kept its campus open to residential students, although it shifted all classes to online instruction. "I think we have a responsibility to our students—who paid to be here, who want to be here, who love it here—to give them the ability to be with their friends, to continue their studies, enjoy the room and board they've already paid for, and to not interrupt their college life," said Liberty president Jerry Falwell, Jr. As one of the only colleges to remain open during the spring of 2020, Liberty came under intense scrutiny, with critics calling Falwell's decision irresponsible and politically motivated. As an outspoken Trump supporter, Falwell downplayed the severity of the pandemic and described measures implemented to protect public health as an "overreaction." "Shame on the media for trying to fan [coronavirus] up and destroy the American economy," he stated. "They're willing to destroy the economy just to hurt Trump"

(Coaston 2020). Although no COVID-19 outbreaks occurred at Liberty before the semester ended in early May, only about 15 percent of students chose to remain on campus after other universities closed.

Institutions of higher learning generally made the transition to online classes more smoothly than K–12 school districts, so most college students managed to finish the 2020 academic year remotely after their campuses closed. Nevertheless, many college students expressed frustration with the loss of face-to-face instruction, classroom discussions, group projects, networking opportunities, social activities, and other valued elements of the residential college experience. They resented paying high tuition rates for online classes that no longer provided access to the professors, facilities, and sense of community they enjoyed on campus. As one New York University student put it in an online petition, "Zoom university is not worth 50K a year" (Kerr 2020). Although many institutions issued students partial refunds for the unused portion of room and board costs, parking fees, and athletic tickets, few offered to discount or refund tuition payments. Administrators cited the cost of transitioning to online instruction and the anticipated drop in state education funding as factors in their refusal to lower tuition.

Dissatisfaction with remote learning, coupled with uncertainty about the impact of COVID-19 on the fall semester, caused many students to rethink their college plans. In a July 2020 survey, 40 percent of prospective first-year undergraduate students reported that the pandemic made them consider changing where or whether they attended college (Quintana 2020). Some analysts predicted an overall decline in college enrollment of 15 to 20 percent if campuses remained closed and classes continued to be conducted online during the fall term. For institutions of higher learning, the prospect of decreased enrollment held severe financial repercussions. Since tuition and fees accounted for more than one-fourth of revenue at public universities and more than one-third of revenue at private colleges, a 20 percent decline in tuition income translated to a loss of $19 billion (Kim et al. 2020). Moreover, institutions stood to lose billions more in room and board payments, bookstore purchases, and athletic proceeds if students did not return to campus in the fall. "The sad fact is that many colleges are racing toward a financial cliff," said Terry Hartle of the American Council on Education (Quintana 2020).

Critics argued that financial considerations should not factor into college administrators' decision-making processes as far as reopening residence halls and offering in-person classes. Instead, they insisted that the health and safety of students, faculty, staff, and the wider community should be the primary considerations. At some universities, groups representing

students, parents, graduate teaching assistants, or local residents organized protests against reopening plans, claiming that they posed too great
a risk to public health. Demonstrators asserted that thousands of college
students returning to campus after months of inactivity, living close
together in dormitories, and socializing without restraint at bars and
house parties created an environment ripe for COVID-19 transmission.
"College kids are college kids," said Carlos del Rio, associate dean of the
Emory University School of Medicine. "That's what I always tell every
university president I talk to: You can make all the plans you want, but at
the end of the day, it's what happens outside your plans that matters"
(Lopez 2020).

Despite the risks, hundreds of colleges nationwide announced plans
to welcome students back to campus in the late summer of 2020. Marie
Lynn Miranda, provost of the University of Notre Dame, argued that institutions of higher learning had an obligation to fulfill their educational
mission. "Education is critical to our democracy," she stated. "When we
can make it happen, we should make it happen" (Quintana 2020). A poll
of 3,000 colleges and universities conducted for the *Chronicle of Higher
Education* found that 27 percent offered classes fully or primarily in person, 44 percent offered classes fully or primarily online, and 21 percent
adopted a hybrid model. College administrators acknowledged that successful reopening depended on the degree to which students followed the
protocols established to prevent the spread of COVID-19. Public health
experts predicted that coronavirus outbreaks would force many reopened
institutions to restrict student activities on campus or even shut down
again. "They need to be ready to have online classes from their dorm room
and all their meals delivered in boxes," said Davidson College professor
Chris Marsicano (Quintana 2020).

In addition to the measures adopted by K–12 school districts—such
as limiting classroom capacity, increasing distance between desks, and
requiring face masks—many colleges and universities conducted extensive coronavirus testing regimens before reopening their campuses and
dormitories. Notre Dame mailed out more than 12,000 home test kits to
incoming students, for instance, and received a positive rate of less than
1 percent (Quintana 2020). Many schools also attempted to ban parties,
or at least urged students not to attend large social gatherings, at the risk
of incurring disciplinary action or being sent home. Nevertheless, many
institutions that initially reopened their campuses had to revert back to
online instruction following COVID-19 outbreaks in student housing.
After recording around 1,800 cases among students and faculty during
the fall semester, for instance, the University of Michigan closed its dormitories and shifted its 31,000 undergraduate students to remote

instruction for the winter term. "The pandemic hasn't gone away, COVID-19 case numbers continue to increase in Michigan and around the nation, and the winter will bring new and likely greater challenges," said university president Mark Schissel. "Cold and flu season, colder weather, and 'COVID fatigue' present very real obstacles for us. I join all of you in wishing that our winter term could be normal" (French 2020).

Further Reading

CDC. 2020. "The Importance of Reopening America's Schools This Fall." U.S. Department of Health and Human Services, July 23, 2020. https://www.cdc.gov/coronavirus/2019-ncov/community/schools-childcare/reopening-schools.html.

Coaston, Jane. 2020. "Liberty University's Choice to Stay Open during Coronavirus, Explained." Vox, March 25, 2020. https://www.vox.com/2020/3/25/21192712/liberty-university-trump-coronavirus-falwell.

Collinson, Stephen. 2020. "Trump Ignores Recent Calamities in His Push to Reopen Schools." CNN, July 8, 2020. https://www.cnn.com/2020/07/08/politics/donald-trump-schools-coronavirus-education/index.html.

"The Coronavirus Spring: The Historic Closing of U.S. Schools." 2020. *Education Week,* July 1, 2020. https://www.edweek.org/ew/section/multimedia/the-coronavirus-spring-the-historic-closing-of.html.

French, Ron. 2020. "COVID Spurs University of Michigan to Close Dorms, Ask Students to Stay Home." Bridge Michigan, November 6, 2020. https://www.bridgemi.com/talent-education/covid-spurs-university-michigan-close-dorms-ask-students-stay-home.

"Here's Our List of Colleges' Reopening Models." *Chronicle of Higher Education,* October 1, 2020. https://www.chronicle.com/article/heres-a-list-of-colleges-plans-for-reopening-in-the-fall/.

Kerr, Emma. 2020. "Why Students Are Seeking Refunds during COVID-19." *U.S. News and World Report,* April 22, 2020. https://www.usnews.com/education/best-colleges/paying-for-college/articles/college-tuition-refunds-discounts-an-uphill-battle-amid-coronavirus?rec-type=sailthru.

Kim, Hayoung, Charag Krishnan, Jonathan Law, and Ted Rounsaville. 2020. "COVID-19 and U.S. Higher Education Enrollment: Preparing Leaders for Fall." McKinsey and Company, May 21, 2020. https://www.mckinsey.com/industries/public-and-social-sector/our-insights/covid-19-and-us-higher-education-enrollment-preparing-leaders-for-fall#.

Klein, Betsy, and Adam Liptak. 2020. "Trump Trashes CDC School-Reopening Guidelines—Then CDC Updates Them." CNN, July 8, 2020. https://www.cnn.com/2020/07/08/politics/trump-cdc-school-guidelines-funding/index.html.

Lopez, German. 2020. "Experts Say COVID-19 Cases Are Likely about to Surge." Vox, October 5, 2020. https://www.vox.com/future-perfect/2020/9/28/21451436/covid-19-coronavirus-pandemic-fall-winter-third-wave.

North, Anna. 2020. "We Need to Talk about What School Closures Mean for Kids with Disabilities." Vox, August 6, 2020. https://www.vox.com/2020/8/6/21353154/schools-reopening-covid-19-special-education-disabilities.

Parshley, Lois. 2020. "'This Is Exactly What We've Been Warning About': Why Some School Reopenings Have Backfired." Vox, August 17, 2020. https://www.vox.com/2020/8/17/21371822/covid-19-prevention-kids-georgia-mississippi-texas.

Quintana, Chris. 2020. "COVID-19 Will Hit Colleges When Students Arrive for Fall Semester. So Why Open at All? Money Is a Factor." *USA Today,* August 17, 2020. https://www.usatoday.com/story/news/education/2020/08/17/covid-cases-college-fall-semester-tuition/5591245002/.

Schleicher, Andreas. 2020. "The Impact of COVID-19 on Education." Organisation for Economic Co-operation and Development, 2020. https://www.oecd.org/education/the-impact-of-covid-19-on-education-insights-education-at-a-glance-2020.pdf.

Schweigershausen, Erica. 2020. "What's Going on with School Reopenings?" *The Cut,* September 29, 2020. https://www.thecut.com/2020/09/will-schools-open-in-the-fall-reopening-statuses-explained.html.

Politics and Partisanship

To contain the coronavirus pandemic effectively, according to public health experts, the United States required a unified national strategy based on scientific evidence and a collective public response guided by accurate information. Instead, surveys showed that politics and partisanship played a major role in determining state and federal COVID-19 policies—such as stay-at-home orders and timelines for economic reopening—as well as in shaping public attitudes and behavior. In a Pew Research Center poll conducted in June 2020, for instance, 73 percent of Democrats said the actions of ordinary Americans had a great deal of impact on the spread of COVID-19, compared to 44 percent of Republicans. Similarly, 61 percent of Republicans said the country had already overcome the worst of the coronavirus crisis, while 76 percent of Democrats said the worst was yet to come (Doherty 2020).

Polarization based on partisan affiliation affected the degree of public compliance with such recommendations as mask wearing and social distancing, with Democrats overwhelmingly supporting these measures and Republicans—led by President Donald Trump's example—largely opposing them. In fact, protective masks emerged as a symbol of political allegiance for many Americans. Combined with misinformation spread through media outlets and social media, critics charged that staunch partisanship undermined the U.S. coronavirus response at the expense of the nation's public and economic health. "The national conversation about how we behave during this pandemic has been so colored by the partisan divide that it's becoming impossible to talk rationally about the risks we are and are not willing to tolerate," said Boston University epidemiologist Sandro Galea. "If both sides were pushed out of their corners, they would both have to concede quite a bit, and we'd frankly all be safer" (Thomson-DeVeaux 2020).

Politics Guides U.S. Pandemic Response

When COVID-19 outbreaks first threatened the United States in early 2020, many analysts predicted that the global pandemic would bring the American people together in a common cause. They envisioned citizens rising to the occasion of a national crisis and willingly making sacrifices in a patriotic effort to defeat the coronavirus and protect vulnerable members of the community. Even though the country had exhibited extreme political division during the first three years of Trump's presidency, some observers pointed to such earlier events as the terrorist attacks of September 11, 2001, as examples of American resilience and solidarity in response to national challenges.

A *Washington Post* survey conducted in mid-April 2020—when nearly all states had coronavirus restrictions in place—found that more than 90 percent of Democrats and 75 percent of Republicans supported such measures as universal testing, contact tracing, mask wearing, and social distancing to "flatten the curve" of COVID-19 cases nationwide. The researchers noted that political leaders had an opportunity to solidify public opinion and gain widespread compliance by emphasizing their own support for these measures. "Citizens across party lines may be willing to follow expert guidance—even if they may have to sacrifice some privacy—depending on their political leaders' signals," they wrote. "If both parties' leaders encourage citizens to accept expert public health recommendations and measures that have saved lives elsewhere, more lives may well be saved" (Christiani et al. 2020). Instead, Republican and Democratic leaders adopted opposite approaches to the pandemic response.

Faced with high unemployment, low consumer spending, and other indications of a severe economic downturn brought on by the coronavirus lockdowns, Trump downplayed the severity of COVID-19, insisted that the virus would disappear by summer, and pressured states to lift restrictions and reopen their economies by Easter. He also questioned the protective value of face masks, refused to wear them during public appearances, and mocked political rivals for wearing them. During his daily appearances at White House Coronavirus Task Force briefings, Trump dismissed the warnings of medical experts, touted unproven miracle cures, and criticized governors who extended lockdown orders. Public health officials asserted that Trump's rejection of basic coronavirus safety precautions influenced the attitudes of his Republican base. "Whether it is his intention or not, the consequence is that he's undermining scientific authority, trust in science, and trust in scientists," said Harvard University public health professor K. "Vish" Viswanath. "In times of crises, especially public health crises, you want to encourage people to work together in a cooperative way. But he is questioning the advice of his own scientific experts" (Pazzanesse 2020).

Democratic leaders, on the other hand, adopted a more cautious stance. They endorsed stay-at-home orders, school closures, and shutdowns of nonessential businesses as necessary measures to contain the spread of the coronavirus. Even as anti-lockdown protests erupted in many states, Democratic governors expressed determination to keep restrictions in place until new COVID-19 cases dropped to low levels and comprehensive test-and-trace protocols became available to prevent further outbreaks. Many prominent Democrats also embraced and promoted mask wearing and social distancing. Democratic presidential nominee Joe Biden, for instance, rarely appeared in public without a mask throughout his 2020 campaign. "A mask is not a political statement," he declared. "It doesn't matter your party, your point of view. We can save tens of thousands of lives if everyone would just wear a mask for the next few months. Not Democrat or Republican lives, American lives" (Biden 2020).

Media coverage of the pandemic response also diverged on the basis of partisan affiliation. A survey conducted in March 2020 found that viewers who relied on the cable network MSNBC as their main source of political news—more than 90 percent of whom identified with or leaned toward the Democratic Party—were far more likely to answer factual questions about the coronavirus correctly than viewers who relied on Fox News—more than 90 percent of whom identified with or leaned toward the Republican Party (Jurkowitz and Mitchell 2020). People who cited social media as their main source of news, meanwhile, were most likely to be exposed to false or misleading information about the pandemic. Public health experts blamed misinformation for sowing doubt about scientific data and contributing to noncompliance with safety recommendations. One study identified Trump as the source of 38 percent of widely circulated erroneous statements and conspiracy theories. "The president of the United States was the single largest driver of misinformation around COVID," said Cornell University researcher Sarah Evanega. "That's concerning in that there are real-world dire health implications" (Stolberg and Weiland 2020).

Partisan views of the coronavirus crisis espoused by politicians and disseminated through the media led to increasing polarization of public attitudes and behavior. A Brookings Institution analysis found that party affiliation played a more influential role than age, health status, or local infection rates in determining an individual's level of fear about COVID-19 and degree of compliance with mask wearing, social distancing, and other precautions. Likewise, the partisan orientation of state officials largely determined the extent and duration of stay-at-home orders, school closures, mask mandates, and other coronavirus response policies. "At some point, the pandemic and associated media coverage became yet another deeply divisive political issue—a board for politicians to score points on, rather than a challenge for the nation to rise to," the Brookings scholars wrote. "Speeches, tweets, and news coverage became dedicated to giving or taking away points. In an alternative universe, leaders from both parties might have set aside their usual differences, united behind a national strategy, and held each other accountable to implementing it" (Rothwell and Makridis 2020).

While Democrats tended to trust the coronavirus guidelines issued by the U.S. Centers for Disease Control and Prevention (CDC) and state and local health departments, Republicans tended to express more skepticism about mask mandates and other government-imposed restrictions on individual rights and liberties. Despite such differences in attitudes, researchers observed a much narrower partisan gap in people's behavior. In a survey conducted in early July, for instance, 88 percent of Republicans reported that they wore a mask in public (Thomson-DeVeaux 2020). "The evidence we have indicates that most people have tried to be responsible and adopt the recommended behaviors, even at a time of immense polarization and confusion and discomfort," Galea said. "But that doesn't mean we should give politicians a pass for turning these serious, serious health conversations into a political football, because that is very much to our detriment" (Thomson-DeVeaux 2020).

Some observers attributed the reduced political polarization in behavior to self-preservation, as a second wave of coronavirus outbreaks swept through Republican-controlled states that reopened early, such as Arizona, Florida, and Texas. "When people are afraid of getting sick, they rely less on partisan shortcuts and take positions and actions to reduce the risk of what they fear," according to researchers Marc J. Hetherington and Isaac D. Mehlhaff (2020). "Fear of becoming seriously ill from COVID-19 helps blunt knee-jerk partisan reactions, which suggests the most effective public messaging strategy to bring Americans together might be fear itself."

Coronavirus Concerns and the 2020 Election

In the fall of 2020—as businesses reopened, students returned to school, and colder weather drove people indoors—the United States experienced a major resurgence of the coronavirus. As the November 2020 election approached, the nation recorded COVID-19 infection rates of over 100,000 per day and neared 10 million total cases and 250,000 deaths. Concern about the coronavirus and its economic impact emerged as a key issue for millions of voters in the presidential election. Pollster Whit Ayres described the pandemic as the "single most important issue facing the electorate, the one most responsible for the recession, the [disruption] of our educational system, and the disruption of our sports and entertainment life" (Nazaryan 2020).

Once again, however, surveys revealed major partisan differences in voters' assessments of the pandemic response as a factor in the election. In an October Pew Research Center poll, 82 percent of Biden supporters ranked the coronavirus crisis as a "very important" voting issue, compared to 24 percent of Trump supporters. The poll also found that more than two-thirds of Republican voters said the Trump administration had controlled the pandemic "as much as it could have," while only 11 percent of Democratic voters agreed (Karma 2020). Republican views reflected the president's repeated assertions that his administration did a "phenomenal" job responding to the coronavirus outbreak, that the media exaggerated the threat of COVID-19 to hurt his chances for reelection, and that the nation needed to focus on economic recovery. "All they want to talk about is COVID," Trump tweeted. "The Fake News Media is riding COVID, COVID, COVID, all the way to the Election" (Nazaryan 2020).

In the closing weeks of the campaign, Trump held a series of rallies in various states. News footage of these events showed thousands of his supporters crowded close together, with few people observing social-distancing recommendations or wearing masks. In October, Trump announced that he had contracted COVID-19, along with First Lady Melania Trump and several White House advisers. The president spent a weekend undergoing treatment at Walter Reed Medical Center in Washington, DC. After recovering, he continued to insist that Americans should not worry about the coronavirus. "Don't be afraid of COVID," he tweeted. "Don't let it dominate your life" (Nazaryan 2020).

In the end, Trump's reassurances failed to resonate with independent voters, and dissatisfaction with his response to the pandemic contributed to the end of his presidency. A poll conducted in seven key swing states found that 56 percent of voters who shifted their support to Biden in 2020 after voting for Trump in 2016 cited the president's handling of the pandemic as a major factor in their decision. Likewise, 15 percent of undecided voters in a nationwide survey described the coronavirus response as the most important issue in the election (Karma 2020). "Americans rejected Trump's haphazard, inattentive handling of the crisis," one analyst noted. "Much as they are exhausted by public health measures, much as they dread another round of lockdowns, they put their faith in a man [Biden] who has promised a clear and consistent strategy to defeat the disease" (Nazaryan 2020).

Further Reading

Biden, Joe. 2020. "President-Elect Biden Delivers Remarks on COVID-19." C-SPAN, November 9, 2020. https://www.c-span.org/video/?477936-1/president -elect-biden-welcomes-pfizer-vaccine-news-warns-growing-virus-threat.

Christiani, Leah, Marc J. Hetherington, Michael MacKuen, Graeme Robertson, and Emily Wager. 2020. "To Fight the Coronavirus, Most Americans Support Universal Testing and Mandatory Quarantines." *Washington Post,* May 15, 2020. https://www.washingtonpost.com/politics/2020/05 /15/fight-coronavirus-most-americans-support-universal-testing -mandatory-quarantines/.

Doherty, Carroll. 2020. "Republicans, Democrats Move Even Further Apart in Coronavirus Concerns." Pew Research Center, June 25, 2020. https:// www.pewresearch.org/politics/2020/06/25/republicans-democrats -move-even-further-apart-in-coronavirus-concerns/.

Hetherington, Marc J., and Isaac D. Mehlhaff. 2020. "American Attitudes toward COVID-19 Are Divided by Party. The Pandemic Itself Might Undo That." *Washington Post,* August 18, 2020. https://www.washingtonpost.com /politics/2020/08/18/american-attitudes-toward-covid-19-are-divided -by-party-pandemic-itself-might-undo-that/.

Jurkowitz, Mark, and Amy Mitchell. 2020. "Cable TV and COVID-19." Pew Research Center, April 1, 2020. https://www.journalism.org/2020/04/01 /cable-tv-and-covid-19-how-americans-perceive-the-outbreak-and-view -media-coverage-differ-by-main-news-source/.

Karma, Roge. 2020. "Poll: The Majority of Trump Voters Don't See COVID-19 as an Important Election Issue." Vox, October 25, 2020. https://www.vox.com /2020/10/25/21532166/pew-poll-republicans-democrats-coronavirus-issue -election-economy-polarization.

Nazaryan, Alexander. 2020. "How Trump Fumbled the Coronavirus Crisis and Sabotaged His Own Reelection." Yahoo! News, November 9, 2020. https://www.yahoo.com/now/how-trump-fumbled-the-coronavirus-crisis-and-sabotaged-his-own-reelection-190428870.html.

Pazzanesse, Christina. 2020. "Calculating Possible Fallout of Trump's Dismissal of Face Masks." *Harvard Gazette,* October 27, 2020. https://news.harvard.edu/gazette/story/2020/10/possible-fallout-from-trumps-dismissal-of-face-masks/.

Rothwell, Jonathan, and Christos Makridis. 2020. "Politics Is Wrecking America's Pandemic Response." Brookings Institution, September 17, 2020. https://www.brookings.edu/blog/up-front/2020/09/17/politics-is-wrecking-americas-pandemic-response/.

Stolberg, Sheryl Gay, and Noah Weiland. 2020. "Study Finds 'Single Largest Driver' of Coronavirus Misinformation: Trump." *New York Times,* October 22, 2020. https://www.nytimes.com/2020/09/30/us/politics/trump-coronavirus-misinformation.html.

Thomson-DeVeaux, Amelia. 2020. "Republicans and Democrats See COVID-19 Very Differently. Is That Making People Sick?" FiveThirtyEight, July 23, 2020. https://fivethirtyeight.com/features/republicans-and-democrats-see-covid-19-very-differently-is-that-making-people-sick/.

CHAPTER FOUR

Profiles

This chapter provides illuminating biographical profiles of important figures in the development and implementation of the Trump administration's pandemic response—including White House Coronavirus Task Force members Deborah Birx and Anthony Fauci—as well as Democratic governors whose aggressive state responses brought them into conflict with the president, such as Andrew Cuomo of New York and Gretchen Whitmer of Michigan.

Deborah Birx (1956–)

Response coordinator for the White House Coronavirus Task Force

Deborah Leah Birx was born in Pennsylvania on April 4, 1956. She was the youngest of three children born to Donald Birx, who worked as a mathematician and electrical engineer, and Adele Sparks Birx, who taught nursing. Birx was a bright, curious child who became interested in science at an early age. She and her two older brothers turned their backyard shed into a laboratory where they conducted experiments and invented contraptions, such as a satellite antenna that caught signals by moving around on roller skates. "We were allowed to run free with all our experimentation," her brother Don recalled. "Whether it was astronomy, geology, biology—anything we'd want to get into, we were given a lot of flexibility and freedom to do it" (Paul 2020).

During her high school years, Birx enjoyed entering projects in science competitions. As a sophomore at Lampeter-Strasburg High School, she took third prize in the Lancaster City-County Science Fair and received a write-up in the local newspaper. As a junior at Carlisle High School, Birx competed in the 1973 International Science and Engineering Fair (ISEF) in San Diego—an annual event featuring 1,500 students from around 70 countries who must qualify by winning regional science fairs. Her project on fossils, entitled *Paleobotany in Reference to the Carboniferous Period*, received third place in the Earth and Space Sciences category and won awards from the U.S. Army and Navy. During her senior year, Birx won the grand prize at the Capital Area Science Fair.

Birx went on to attend Houghton College in New York, earning a bachelor's degree in chemistry in 1976. That same year, she married Paige Reffe, an attorney specializing in international law who served as an "advance man" planning overseas trips for President Bill Clinton. The marriage produced two children. In 1980, Birx received her medical degree from the Hershey School of Medicine at Penn State University. She then became an active duty reserve officer in the U.S. Army and continued her medical training by serving a two-year residency in internal medicine at the Walter Reed Army Medical Center and fellowships in basic and clinical immunology at the National Institutes of Health (NIH) in Bethesda, Maryland. In 1985, Birx launched her career with the Department of Defense as a U.S. Army physician specializing in immunology. She eventually achieved the rank of colonel and received two U.S. Meritorious Service Medals and the Legion of Merit award for her leadership skills and research accomplishments.

In the early 1980s, a mysterious, deadly disease began appearing in otherwise healthy gay men. It attacked their immune systems and left them vulnerable to opportunistic infections, including rare forms of pneumonia and cancer. Doctors called the disease Acquired Immune Deficiency Syndrome (AIDS) and identified Human Immunodeficiency Virus (HIV) as the pathogen responsible. As the AIDS epidemic spread and claimed thousands of lives, Birx's research focused on developing a vaccine to prevent the transmission of HIV. She recalled the early years of the AIDS crisis as particularly frustrating. "When you're trained in medicine and it's the '80s and you've got all this hi-tech stuff and this ability to diagnose everything, when you not only couldn't make a diagnosis, you didn't know what the problem was, and you didn't know how to treat it, it was devastating, it was incredibly humbling," she stated (Srikanth 2020).

Birx spent 16 years of her career conducting research toward a vaccine for HIV. In 1996, she became director of the U.S. Military HIV Research Program at the Walter Reed Army Institute of Research. In that role, she oversaw clinical trials of the first vaccine that effectively lowered the risk of contracting HIV. Birx remembered being inspired to work harder by the honor and sacrifice demonstrated by the soldiers she treated for AIDS. "They died with such courage and such willingness to try different things, realizing it may not help them, but it would help the person behind them," she said. "I just never saw that level of altruism, amidst just death and despair, from the patients themselves" (Holpuch 2020).

In 2003, the George W. Bush administration announced the creation of the President's Emergency Plan for AIDS Relief (PEPFAR), an international public health initiative intended to make life-saving HIV therapies available to people in developing countries. Birx, who had been working on vaccine research in Kenya, immediately returned to the United States to express her support for the program. She prepared a 180-slide Power-Point presentation and spent days waiting outside the home of Joe O'Neill, the director of the Office of National AIDS policy, to make her case. In 2005, Birx became director of the global HIV/AIDS division at the U.S. Centers for Disease Control and Prevention (CDC). She managed an annual budget of $1.5 billion and oversaw the activities of nearly 2,000 staff members working to strengthen local health systems and reduce HIV transmission in countries around the world.

In 2014, President Barack Obama appointed Birx as coordinator of the U.S. Government Activities to Combat HIV/AIDS and U.S. special representative for Global Health Diplomacy, an ambassador-level position within the State Department that placed her in charge of the federal government's programs to prevent the spread of HIV around the world. Birx thus took control of PEPFAR, which saved millions of lives worldwide by increasing global access to anti-AIDS education programs and medications. Birx earned the respect of colleagues by coupling a scientific approach driven by data with a sympathetic touch developed through experience. "She's always tried to bring it down to a connection on more of a personal level," said Jen Kates, director of global health and HIV policy at the Kaiser Family Foundation. "Sometimes she'll talk about her own experience as a parent. Sometimes she'll talk about her experience working 30 years ago in the military and seeing the first HIV cases. But she always does try to make that connection, and I think that's one of the hallmarks of her leadership" (Beaubien 2020).

In early 2020, a new threat to global public health emerged in the form of a novel coronavirus, SARS-CoV-2. The pathogen first infected humans in China, causing a respiratory illness called COVID-19, and quickly spread around the world. Shortly after the first U.S. case appeared in January, President Donald Trump formed the White House Coronavirus Task Force to oversee the federal government's response to the emerging pandemic. On February 26, Trump named Vice President Mike Pence as chairman of the task force, taking over the role originally performed by Secretary of Health and Human Services Alex Azar. The president also appointed Birx to the task force in the position of coronavirus response coordinator. Although the leadership hierarchy of the group initially caused some confusion, Trump later clarified that Birx reported to Pence, who described the doctor as his "right arm" (Srikanth 2020).

The White House issued a statement announcing Birx's appointment to the task force. "Ambassador Birx is a scientist, physician, and mom, with three decades of public health expertise, including virulent diseases, their vaccines, and interagency coordination," it read. "She has been utilizing the best science to change the course of the HIV pandemic and bring the pandemic under control, community by community and country by country" (Pence 2020). Many public health experts praised Birx's addition, citing her expertise in immunology and her experience leading the global fight against an infectious disease. "She is somebody that knows how to manage the whole of the U.S. government to move it toward a particular goal," said Georgetown University global health policy expert Matthew Kavanaugh. "If the White House lets her do that, it could be exactly the kind of coordination that has been lacking up to this point" (Srikanth 2020). "When it is a matter of making tough decisions, she will do it," added Emory University global health professor Carlos del Rio. "And that, to me, is what we need right now" (Holpuch 2020).

On March 16, the coronavirus task force began holding daily press briefings at the White House. Trump usually opened each news conference by reading a prepared statement updating the media and the American people on the latest developments. Birx—one of only two women in the group, which by then included 22 members—often stood behind the podium with Pence and other officials involved in the federal pandemic response, including her colleague Dr. Anthony Fauci, director of the National Institute of Allergy and Infectious Diseases. In the midst of powerful men wearing business suits or military dress uniforms, Birx stood out in plain shirt dresses accented with colorful, patterned silk scarves. She explained that she developed this signature style to simplify packing when she traveled internationally as a global health ambassador. Many viewers found her feminine presence reassuring, and some admirers began posting photos of themselves wearing scarves on social media. "Birx's style speaks to her emotional intelligence," wrote *Washington Post* fashion critic Robin Givhan. "While the regular briefings are filled with folks in suits and uniforms—clipboard types who are very good at going through the motions of competence—Birx makes one feel like she'd be the one willing to put a cool compress to a fevered brow while everyone else was backing out of the room" (Srikanth 2020).

During the briefings, Birx and other task force members often stepped up to the microphone to make presentations, discuss specific issues, or answer questions from the press. Birx often used personal stories to reinforce her message about the importance of washing hands, wearing face coverings, social distancing, and staying home to prevent the spread of SARS-CoV-2. She targeted her message at young Americans, warning that they could carry the virus without experiencing symptoms and transmit it to more vulnerable populations. To prove her point, she told a story about her grandmother, who was 11 years old during the 1918 influenza pandemic that killed an estimated 50 million people worldwide. The child unknowingly brought the virus home and infected her mother, who ended up dying from the disease. "I can tell you my grandmother lived with that for 88 years," Birx said. "This is the message that is important to everybody. This is not a theoretic. This is a reality. You can see the number of deaths that are occurring. We all have a role in preventing them" (Beaubien 2020).

In addition to admonishing the public to take precautions against the coronavirus, Birx also echoed some of the Trump administration's reassurances about the nation's ability to contain it. On March 26, as reports emerged about hospitals in New York City being overwhelmed with COVID-19 patients and experiencing shortages of beds, ventilators, and protective equipment, Birx insisted that the situation was under control and urged people not to panic. "There is no situation in the United States right now that warrants that kind of discussion," she stated. "To say that to the American people, to make the implication that when they need a hospital bed, it's not going to be there, or when they need that ventilator, it's not going to be there, we don't have evidence of that right now" (Schwartz 2020). Harvard University epidemiologist Marc Lipsitch rejected Birx's assessment of the situation, calling it "rosy" and "deceptive" (Beaubien 2020).

Many viewers appreciated the way Birx alternated between providing scientific facts and offering heartfelt reassurances. "Her appearances are a cross between a war briefing and FDR's fireside chats," said NPR correspondent Jason Beaubien (2020). "She mixes the minutiae of disease transmission with deeply personal stories, then pivots to complex discussions of antibody testing for the virus. She scolds and reassures within minutes of each other." Yet some critics asserted that, as a public health expert, Birx had a responsibility to set the record straight when Trump or other administration officials made false or misleading statements in their eagerness to downplay the severity of the crisis and reopen the U.S.

economy. Instead, the job of correcting misstatements made in task force briefings usually fell to Fauci.

During one controversial news conference on April 24, for instance, Trump proposed using ultraviolet light or chemical disinfectants inside the human body to kill the coronavirus—ideas that many medical experts rejected as dangerous. Although Birx appeared visibly shaken by the president's suggestion in a video clip that went viral, she did not express any objection. Later, she defended Trump's statement by saying he was merely digesting information by musing about it out loud. Supporters attributed Birx's task force performance to years of building political coalitions to tackle public health problems. "Her goal is to focus on the science and work across political boundaries and pull people together," her brother explained. "She's learned over the years that if you are going to solve a complex problem, like HIV or the new coronavirus, you really need everyone working together as a team and have the cooperation, respect, and ability to engage people who are on different ends of the political spectrum" (Paul 2020).

Further Reading

Beaubien, Jason. 2020. "A Leading Voice on the Coronavirus Task Force, Deborah Birx Draws Praise and Criticism." NPR, March 27, 2020. https://www.npr.org/sections/health-shots/2020/03/27/822346158/a-leading-voice-on-coronavirus-task-force-deborah-birx-draws-praise-and-criticis.

"Deborah L. Birx, M.D." 2020. U.S. Department of State. https://www.state.gov/biographies/deborah-l-birx-md/.

Holpuch, Amanda. 2020. "She's a Legend in the Fight against HIV. Now Dr. Deborah Birx Is Taking on COVID-19." *Guardian,* March 13, 2020. https://www.theguardian.com/world/2020/mar/12/coronavirus-dr-deborah-birx-hiv-aids.

Paul, Aparna. 2020. "From ISEF to the White House, Dr. Deborah Birx Leads the Country during a Health Crisis." Society for Science and the Public, March 23, 2020. https://www.societyforscience.org/blog/from-isef-to-the-white-house-dr-deborah-birx-leads-the-country-during-a-public-health-crisis/.

Pence, Mike. 2020. "Vice President Pence Announces Ambassador Debbie Birx to Serve as the White House Coronavirus Response Coordinator." The White House, February 27, 2020. https://www.whitehouse.gov/briefings-statements/vice-president-pence-announces-ambassador-debbie-birx-serve-white-house-coronavirus-response-coordinator/.

Pesce, Nicole Lyn. 2020. "Who Is Deborah Birx, the Doctor Whose Reaction When Trump Suggested People Should Inject Disinfectants Has Gone Viral?" MarketWatch, April 24, 2020. https://www.marketwatch.com

/story/who-is-deborah-birx-the-doctor-whose-reaction-when-trump
-suggested-people-inject-disinfectants-has-gone-viral-2020-04-24.

Schwartz, Ian. 2020. *"Dr. Birx: Coronavirus Data Doesn't Match the Doomsday
Media Predictions." Real Clear Politics, March 26, 2020.* https://www.real
clearpolitics.com/video/2020/03/26/dr_birx_coronavirus_data_doesnt
_match_the_doomsday_media_predictions_or_analysis.html.

Srikanth, Anagha. 2020. "Who Is Coronavirus Warrior Dr. Deborah Birx?" *The
Hill,* March 26, 2020. https://thehill.com/changing-america/well-being
/prevention-cures/489717-who-is-coronavirus-warrior-dr-deborah-birx.

Andrew Cuomo (1957–)

Governor of New York during the COVID-19 pandemic

Andrew Mark Cuomo was born on December 6, 1957, in New York City. He was the second of five children born to Mario Cuomo, a politician who served as governor of New York from 1983 to 1994, and Matilda Raffa Cuomo, an educator and mentoring advocate. Andrew's younger brother, Chris Cuomo, became a national news anchor and analyst. Andrew grew up in Queens as part of an extended family of hard-working Italian immigrants. He attended Archbishop Molloy High School, graduating in 1975, and went on to earn a bachelor's degree from Fordham University in the Bronx in 1979. Three years later, Cuomo received his law degree from the University of Albany.

Cuomo first became involved in politics in 1982, when he served as the manager of his father's successful campaign to become the 52nd governor of New York. He remained one of the administration's top advisers throughout Mario Cuomo's three terms in office. Meanwhile, the younger Cuomo launched his own career as a lawyer and public servant. In 1984, he became an assistant district attorney for Manhattan. Two years later, he founded a nonprofit organization called Housing Enterprise for the Less Privileged (HELP), which built and operated transitional and low-income housing to alleviate the problem of homelessness in New York City.

Cuomo married Kerry Kennedy, the daughter of former U.S. senator and attorney general Robert F. Kennedy, in 1990. They had three daughters—Mariah, Cara, and Michaela—before divorcing in 2005. In 1993, shortly after Democrat Bill Clinton became president of the United States, Cuomo joined the U.S. Department of Housing and Urban Development (HUD) as the assistant secretary for community planning and development. Clinton appointed Cuomo secretary of HUD during his second term, and Cuomo held that position from 1997 through 2001.

The following year, Cuomo ran for political office for the first time as a Democratic challenger to Republican George Pataki, who had defeated Cuomo's father to become governor of New York in 1994. During the campaign, Cuomo questioned Pataki's leadership following the terrorist attacks of September 11, 2001, claiming that the governor had "stood behind" New York City mayor Rudolph Giuliani and "held the leader's coat" during the crisis (Lentz 2019). Cuomo came under criticism for politicizing the tragedy and withdrew from the gubernatorial race. After working in a private law practice for several years, Cuomo returned to politics in 2006, when he was elected attorney general for the State of New York. During his tenure, he earned a reputation as reformer who cracked down on government corruption, protected the interests of consumers and taxpayers, challenged discrimination, and enforced environmental laws.

After fellow Democrat Eliot Spitzer resigned in 2008 due to his involvement in a prostitution scandal, Cuomo launched a successful campaign for the office once held by his father. He took office as the 56th governor of New York in 2010 and won reelection in 2014 and 2018. As a vocal supporter of LGBTQ rights, Cuomo signed a law in 2011 making New York one of the earliest states to legalize same-sex marriage. In 2013, Cuomo signed one of the toughest gun control laws in the nation, the New York SAFE Act. The following year, he lent his support to a movement that led to the legalization of medical marijuana in the state.

As governor, Cuomo also assisted working families by increasing the state minimum wage to $15 per hour, establishing a paid family leave program, investing in public education, and providing free college tuition for students from low- and middle-income families. In the realm of environmental protection, Cuomo approved a state ban on the controversial oil and gas extraction method known as hydraulic fracturing or fracking, and he joined other states in pledging to continue following the Paris Climate Accords after President Donald Trump withdrew the United States from the agreement.

In 2020, a highly transmissible new coronavirus emerged in China and quickly spread around the world. As a major international travel hub with high population density, New York City became the epicenter of the pandemic in the United States. From the time public health officials confirmed New York's first COVID-19 case on March 1, the number of cases exploded to exceed 80,000 by the end of the month. Cuomo took initial steps to prepare for the crisis on March 3, when he authorized $40 million in state funding for the response. On March 7, he declared a state of emergency and expanded state efforts to procure test kits and personal protective equipment for medical responders. Over the next week, Cuomo implemented a series of restrictions aimed at slowing the spread of the coronavirus, such as closing public schools, postponing the annual St. Patrick's Day parade, canceling Broadway performances, and banning visitors to nursing homes.

On March 15, Cuomo published an open letter in the *New York Times* asking Trump for federal assistance to help states combat the coronavirus. "Every country affected by this crisis has handled it on a national basis," he wrote. "The United States has not. State and local governments alone simply do not have the capacity or resources to do what is necessary, and we don't want a patchwork quilt of policies" (Cuomo 2020). The governor urged the Trump administration to loosen FDA restrictions on testing, establish national standards for enacting stay-at-home orders, and mobilize the military to help states obtain medical supplies and expand hospital capacity.

On March 17, however, Cuomo disputed Mayor Bill de Blasio's warning that New York City's eight million residents should prepare for a lockdown. "There is not going to be any quarantine, no one is going to lock you in your home. No one is going to tell you you can't leave the city. That is not going to happen," Cuomo declared. "That will just cause people to go somewhere else, and that will be counterproductive" (Associated Press 2020). On March 19, when California enacted the first statewide stay-at-home order, Cuomo expressed concern that such drastic measures would cause panic. "In many ways, the fear is more dangerous than the virus," he said (Gold and Robinson 2020).

The continued surge in COVID-19 cases soon convinced Cuomo to rethink his position. On March 22, he issued an executive order called "New York State on PAUSE" that closed all nonessential businesses and required residents to remain at home except to acquire food, access medical care, or exercise outdoors. It also prohibited social gatherings and recommended that individuals maintain 6 feet of distance from others in public spaces. By the time the lockdown order took effect, New York had recorded more than 15,000 COVID-19 cases and 76 deaths.

During New York's shutdown, Cuomo emerged as a leading figure in the U.S. response to the coronavirus crisis. He gave daily televised briefings to provide state residents with up-to-date information on the number of confirmed cases, the availability of testing, and the public health measures recommended to slow the spread of the virus. Cuomo also expressed compassion for families that lost loved ones, concern for people who lost jobs, and empathy for everyone struggling to adjust to the major disruption caused by his stay-at-home order. "I assume full responsibility," he stated. "I know people are upset. I know businesses will be hurt by this. I don't feel good about that. I feel very bad about that because I know we're going to have to deal with that issue as soon as this immediate public health issue is over. But my judgment is do whatever is necessary to contain this virus, and then we will manage the consequences afterwards" (Herbert 2020).

Political analysts praised Cuomo's calm demeanor, clear messaging, and willingness to take responsibility for the well-being of his constituents. Public approval of his leadership during the crisis sent his popularity level skyrocketing, even as New York's death toll rose to 27,500 by May 15—or one-third of all COVID-19 deaths in the United States at that time. As hospitals became overwhelmed by the flood of patients, Cuomo converted convention centers to medical facilities and convinced the federal government to provide ventilators and medical supplies. The governor also extended lockdown restrictions and chastised New Yorkers who resisted doing their part to prevent the virus from spreading. "I don't know what they're not understanding," Cuomo said. "This is not a joke and I am not kidding" (Herbert 2020).

As the daily case counts began to decline, Trump pushed New York and other states to lift social-distancing restrictions and reopen their economies. When Cuomo and other governors called for a more cautious approach, Trump asserted that he had the authority to force states to reopen. Cuomo strenuously objected to the president's claim and declared his intention to follow his own reopening plan. "We don't have a king, we have a president," the governor stated. "If he says to me, 'I declare it open,' and that is a public health risk or it's reckless with the welfare of the people of my state, I will oppose it" (Smith 2020). Cuomo led an alliance of seven East Coast states (Connecticut, Delaware, Massachusetts, New Jersey, New York, and Pennsylvania) that pledged to coordinate their reopening plans and present a united front in the face of Trump's demands.

As New York emerged from the worst of the crisis, Cuomo faced some criticism for the extreme toll the pandemic took on his state. Some critics claimed that he could have prevented thousands of deaths by issuing his stay-at-home order sooner. "There's something disturbing about Cuomo being hailed as the hero of the pandemic when he should rightly be one of the villains," Lyta Gold and Nathan Robinson (2020) wrote in the *Guardian*. "He is now only able to attain praise for his actions because his earlier failures made those actions necessary. He's lauded for addressing a problem that he himself partly caused." Supporters, on the other hand, argued that Cuomo's measured, orderly approach helped ensure public buy-in and prevent panic. They also pointed out only three weeks elapsed between New York's first confirmed COVID-19 case and the governor's shutdown order, compared to two months for California. While Cuomo acknowledged the hardships caused by the pandemic, he expressed optimism for the future. "We're going to be the better for it," he said. "Dealing with hardship actually makes you stronger" (Herbert 2020).

Further Reading

Associated Press. 2020. "Coronavirus in NY: Shelter in Place? Cuomo Disputes de Blasio's Lockdown Warning." Syracuse.com, March 19, 2020. https://www.syracuse.com/coronavirus/2020/03/coronavirus-in-ny-shelter-in -place-cuomo-disputes-de-blasios-lockdown-warning.html.

Axelson, Ben. 2020. "Coronavirus Timeline in NY: Here's How Gov. Cuomo Has Responded to COVID-19 Pandemic since January." Syracuse.com, April 14, 2020. https://www.syracuse.com/coronavirus/2020/04/corona virus-timeline-in-ny-heres-how-gov-cuomo-has-responded-to-covid-19 -pandemic-since-january.html.

Cuomo, Andrew M. 2014. *All Things Possible: Setbacks and Success in Politics and in Life.* New York: HarperCollins.

Cuomo, Andrew M. 2020. "Andrew Cuomo to President Trump: Mobilize the Military to Help Fight Coronavirus." *New York Times,* March 15, 2020. https://www.nytimes.com/2020/03/15/opinion/andrew-cuomo -coronavirus-trump.html.

Gold, Lyta, and Nathan Robinson. 2020. "Andrew Cuomo Is No Hero. He's to Blame for New York's Coronavirus Catastrophe." *Guardian,* May 20, 2020. https://www.theguardian.com/commentisfree/2020/may/20/andrew -cuomo-new-york-coronavirus-catastrophe.

Herbert, Geoff. 2020. "Who Is Andrew Cuomo? About the NY Governor Leading the Coronavirus Response in State." Syracuse.com, March 23, 2020. https://www.syracuse.com/state/2020/03/who-is-andrew-cuomo-about -the-ny-governor-leading-coronavirus-response-in-state.html.

Lentz, Jon. 2019. "Andrew Cuomo's Biggest Gaffes." City and State New York, January 10, 2019. https://www.cityandstateny.com/articles/politics/new -york-state/andrew-cuomos-biggest-gaffes.html.

Shnayerson, Michael. 2015. *The Contender: Andrew Cuomo.* New York: Twelve.

Smith, Allan. 2020. "Trump Backs Down after Cuomo, Other Governors Unite on Coronavirus Response." NBC News, April 14, 2020. https://www .nbcnews.com/politics/donald-trump/trump-backs-down-after-cuomo -governors-unite-coronavirusk-response-n1183471.

Anthony Fauci (1940–)

Director of the National Institute of Allergy and Infectious Diseases

Anthony Stephen Fauci (pronounced FOW-chee) was born on December 24, 1940, in the Brooklyn borough of New York City. His parents, Stephen A. Fauci and Eugenia Abys Fauci, owned a pharmacy in the Dyker Heights neighborhood. Anthony delivered prescriptions on his bicycle, and his older sister, Denise, helped out at the cash register. Like many kids growing up in New York City, Anthony loved baseball. Even though he lived near Ebbets Field—home of the Brooklyn Dodgers—he became a devoted fan of the New York Yankees. "Half the kids in Brooklyn were Yankee fans," he recalled. "We spent our days arguing who was better: Duke Snider versus Mickey Mantle; Roy Campanella versus Yogi Berra; Pee Wee Reese versus Phil Rizzuto and on and on. Those were the days" (Specter 2020).

Fauci grew up Catholic and attended Regis High School, a private, all-male Jesuit school in Manhattan. Although his daily commute involved several subways and buses, he thrived in the school's academically rigorous environment. "We took four years of Greek, four years of Latin, three years of French, ancient history, theology," he remembered. Fauci also served as captain of the school basketball team and once hoped to play professional basketball. "I thought this was what I wanted to do with myself," he acknowledged. "But, being a realist, I very quickly found out that a five-seven, really fast, good-shooting point guard will never be as good as a really fast, good-shooting seven-footer. I decided to change the direction of my career" (Specter 2020).

After graduating from Regis in 1958, Fauci attended the College of the Holy Cross in Worcester, Massachusetts. Four years later, he earned a bachelor's degree in Greek Classics with a concentration in pre-medical studies. Fauci went on to earn his medical degree from Cornell University, graduating first in his class in 1966. "Tony has always been driven," noted his longtime friend Michael Osterholm. "Whatever he was doing, he had to do it better than anybody else. I don't know if it was certainty or something else. But he was meant to lead. Always. Everyone who knew him knew that. And Tony knew it, too" (Specter 2020). Fauci served his residency in internal medicine at New York Presbyterian/Weill Cornell Medicine.

In 1968, Fauci became a clinical research associate at the National Institute of Allergy and Infectious Diseases (NIAID)—one of the 27 research institutes and centers, each focusing on different biomedical and public health disciplines, that comprise the National Institutes of Health (NIH) within the U.S. Department of Health and Human Services. Fauci rose steadily through the ranks until President Ronald Reagan appointed him director of NIAID in 1984. Fauci would remain in that role for 36 years and provide expert advice to six presidents as the nation faced outbreaks of such infectious diseases as HIV, SARS, MERS, influenza, Ebola, and West Nile virus. Fauci reportedly turned down offers to become head of the NIH, preferring instead to oversee NIAID's groundbreaking research into infectious, immunologic, and allergic diseases. He gained a reputation as one of the world's leading experts in his field and ranked among the most-cited contributors to scientific journals.

Fauci's research in the 1970s focused on immunology and diseases relating to the immune system. He investigated a rare condition called vasculitis, for instance, in which an overactive immune system attacks the patient's own blood vessels, causing chronic inflammation, organ damage, and eventually death. Fauci and his colleagues discovered that chemotherapy drugs used to suppress cancerous tumors could also be used to regulate overactive immune systems in vasculitis patients. "I thought if we could somehow give a cancer drug at a low enough dose, perhaps we could turn the disease off," he recalled. "First we did it in a few patients, and, much to our delight, they had a total remission. Before you know it, we ended up curing a very, very lethal, albeit uncommon, disease" (Specter 2020). Fauci and other researchers eventually applied this technique to help patients with lupus, rheumatoid arthritis, and such rare inflammatory diseases as granulomatosis with polyangiitis.

During the 1980s, Fauci's research centered on finding treatments for Acquired Immune Deficiency Syndrome (AIDS), a deadly disease that first appeared among otherwise healthy gay men. His work contributed to scientific knowledge of the Human Immunodeficiency Virus (HIV) and how it destroys the immune system, leaving the body susceptible to opportunistic infections and eventually causing AIDS. After he became director of the NIAID in 1984, Fauci became a target of AIDS activists such as Larry Kramer, who claimed that the Reagan administration failed to take aggressive steps to combat the epidemic. Kramer attacked Fauci relentlessly in the press, blaming him for the federal government's inaction and describing him as an "incompetent idiot" and a "murderer." "God, I hated him," Kramer acknowledged. "As far as I was concerned, he was the central focus of evil in the world" (Specter 2020).

In 1988, a group of angry AIDS protesters marched through the NIH campus in Bethesda, Maryland, demanding faster approval of experimental treatments for HIV. Rather than avoiding confrontation, Fauci invited several of the protest leaders into his office and listened to their perspectives. "There was a feeling in science that doctors know best, scientists know best," Fauci said. "Then, when we dealt with this disease that was brand new—that was frightening, that was killing people in a way that was historic—the people who were impacted by the disease wanted to have something to say about how we conducted research" (Specter 2020). Fauci ended up promoting changes that expanded patients' access to experimental drugs and establishing a division within the NIAID dedicated to HIV and AIDS research. Kramer eventually became a close friend and once described Fauci as "the only true and great hero" among U.S. government officials involved in the AIDS crisis (Specter 2020). Years later, Fauci helped the George W. Bush administration launch the President's Emergency Plan for AIDS Relief (PEPFAR), a global public health program that made life-saving HIV medications available to people in developing countries.

Throughout the 1990s and 2000s, Fauci returned to the spotlight each time the United States faced a threat to public health. He served as an adviser to help presidents determine the best federal response to disease outbreaks, and he served as a media spokesperson to help inform and reassure the American people. "During a health emergency, it's the scientists and physicians that are the credible people to the American public, not politicians," said former Secretary of Health and Human Services Donna Shalala (Grady 2020). Fauci always tried to explain medical facts in a clear, understandable way. "Tony has essentially become the embodiment of the biomedical and public-health research enterprise in the United States," said microbiologist David Relman. "Nobody is a more tireless champion of the truth and the facts" (Specter 2020). Behind the scenes, Fauci also oversaw a $5.9 billion annual budget at the NIAID, where he directed teams of scientists who researched emerging diseases and developed vaccines to limit their impact.

Like many public health experts, Fauci long recommended that the U.S. government take steps to prepare for an infectious disease pandemic. He unsuccessfully sought funding to develop universal "platform" vaccines, for instance, to protect against entire classes of viruses instead of only particular strains. "We keep trying to develop a vaccine for one thing—usually the last one—and it's a waste of time," he explained. Instead, "you could build a chassis for the vaccine, and you would have it on the shelf. Then all you would need to do is insert the gene of the protein you want to express and make a gazillion doses and send it out" (Specter 2020). In 2017, shortly before President Donald Trump took office, Fauci delivered a speech at Georgetown University called "Pandemic Preparedness for the Next Administration." At some point in the future, he predicted, an unknown pathogen would emerge to infect large swaths of humanity. "No matter what, history has told us definitively that it will happen," he asserted (Specter 2020).

In January 2020, therefore, Fauci was not surprised to learn about an unusual outbreak of pneumonia cases in Wuhan, China. "Even before we knew it was a coronavirus, I said it certainly sounds like a coronavirus-SARS type thing," he said. "As soon as it was identified, I called a meeting of top-level people and said, 'Let's start working on a vaccine right now'" (Grady 2020). Fauci recognized that the novel coronavirus, SARS-CoV-2, and the infectious disease it caused in humans, COVID-19, had many qualities that posed a significant public health threat. "You have a random virus jump species from an animal to a human that is spectacularly efficient in spreading from human to human, and has a high degree, relatively speaking, of morbidity and mortality," he noted. "We are living in the perfect storm right now" (Kuchler 2020).

When the Trump administration formed the White House Coronavirus Task Force to oversee the U.S. government's response to the emerging pandemic, Fauci immediately signed on and became one of its most prominent members. In interviews, news briefings, and testimony before Congress, Fauci provided calm, no-nonsense, authoritative assessments of the situation based in medical evidence. *New York Times* writer Denise Grady (2020) described him as the "explainer-in-chief of the coronavirus epidemic." Many Americans appreciated the way Fauci presented facts about the virus, informing them about how it spread and what precautions they could take to minimize their risk of infection. In fact, Fauci gained celebrity status, with his likeness appearing in memes, on bumper stickers, and in the form of a collectible bobblehead. Actor Brad Pitt even portrayed Fauci in a skit for *Saturday Night Live*. Yet the doctor remained humble about his sudden fame. "I believe, in fact I'm certain, that the country, in a very stressful time, needed a symbol of someone who tells the truth, which I do," he stated (Kuchler 2020).

As Trump began participating in the daily task force press briefings, Fauci became the main voice of disagreement when the president downplayed the severity of the virus or made overly optimistic predictions about its impact on American life. If Trump made an inaccurate statement or promoted misinformation, Fauci often managed to correct the record without explicitly saying that the president was wrong. When Trump asserted that COVID-19 cases would disappear with the arrival of warmer spring weather, for instance, Fauci noted that no one knew whether the novel coronavirus would be seasonal since it had only infected humans for a few months. When Trump insisted that a vaccine would be available soon, Fauci offered a more accurate timetable of 12 to 18 months. The two men also disagreed about hydroxychloroquine, a drug used to treat arthritis and malaria, which Trump often touted as a miracle cure for COVID-19. "I say try it," the president stated. "You're not gonna die from this pill" (Specter 2020). Fauci explained that while some anecdotal evidence suggested the drug might be useful, it had not yet been tested using scientific methods and thus could prove ineffective or even dangerous.

Fauci consistently urged Americans to take precautions to prevent the spread of SARS-CoV-2, such as washing hands, wearing face masks, maintaining social distance, and avoiding crowds. Trump frequently ignored Fauci's advice by refusing to wear a mask, scheduling campaign rallies, and pushing to reopen the U.S. economy. A Quinnipiac University poll found that 65 percent of voters trusted the coronavirus information provided by Fauci, compared to only 30 percent who trusted information from the president (Phelps and Gittleson 2020).

Fauci's cautious position came under intense criticism from Trump supporters and conservative media personalities, who tended to discount his expertise and question his recommendations. Critics claimed that Fauci and other scientists exaggerated the threat posed by the coronavirus to disrupt the economic recovery and harm the president's chances for reelection. "Has anyone else noticed that every suggestion by Dr. Doom Fauci just happens to also be the worst possible thing for the economy?" tweeted conservative pundit Bill Mitchell. "That's not an accident folks" (Specter 2020). Several administration officials wrote editorials or social media posts intended to discredit Fauci. Trump contributed to the backlash by retweeting a message with the hashtag #FireFauci. Fauci became the subject of death threats and required a security detail to protect him and his family. He acknowledged that he found the conflict stressful. "I'm an apolitical person," he noted. "It's pretty tough walking a tightrope while trying to get your message out and people are trying to pit you against the president" (Phelps and Gittleson 2020).

The coronavirus task force stopped holding daily press conferences in late April and shifted its emphasis toward reopening the economy. In mid-June, the nation experienced a resurgence of COVID-19 cases in Florida, Texas, Arizona, and California, with daily numbers exceeding earlier totals. Fauci expressed frustration with the situation, which he attributed to people's reluctance to heed the advice of public health authorities. "I think we have to realize that some states jumped ahead of themselves," he noted. "Other states did it correctly, but the citizenry didn't listen to the guidelines and they decided they were going to stay in bars and go to congregations of crowds and celebrations" (Kuchler 2020).

Fauci has received many prestigious awards for his decades of work in public health, including the Presidential Medal of Freedom, the National Medal of Science, and the Mary Woodard Lasker Award for Public Service. In his personal life, he has been married to Christine Grady, a nurse who serves as chief of the Department of Bioethics at the NIH Clinical Center, since 1985. They are the parents of three adult daughters, Jennifer, Megan, and Alison.

Further Reading

"Anthony S. Fauci, M.D." 2020. National Institute of Allergy and Infectious Diseases, February 5, 2020. https://www.niaid.nih.gov/about/anthony-s-fauci-md-bio.

Cohen, Jon. 2020. "'I'm Going to Keep Pushing.' Anthony Fauci Tries to Make the White House Listen to Facts of the Pandemic." *Science,* March 22, 2020. https://www.sciencemag.org/news/2020/03/i-m-going-keep-pushing-anthony-fauci-tries-make-white-house-listen-facts-pandemic.

Grady, Denise. 2020. "Not His First Epidemic: Dr. Anthony Fauci Sticks to the Facts." *New York Times,* March 8, 2020. https://www.nytimes.com/2020/03/08/health/fauci-coronavirus.html.

Kuchler, Hannah. 2020. "Anthony Fauci: 'We Are Living in the Perfect Storm.'" *Financial Times,* July 10, 2020. https://www.ft.com/content/57834c2c-a078-4736-9173-8fb32cfbbf4e.

Phelps, Jordyn, and Ben Gittleson. 2020. "President Donald Trump Meets His Match in Anthony Fauci." ABC News, July 16, 2020. https://abcnews.go.com/Politics/president-donald-trump-meets-match-anthony-fauci-analysis/story?id=71822115.

Specter, Michael. 2020. "How Anthony Fauci Became America's Doctor." *New Yorker,* April 10, 2020. https://www.newyorker.com/magazine/2020/04/20/how-anthony-fauci-became-americas-doctor.

Mike Pence (1959–)

Vice president of the United States and chairman of the White House Coronavirus Task Force

Michael Richard Pence was born on June 7, 1959, in Columbus, Indiana. He grew up as one of six children in an Irish Catholic family. His parents, Edward Pence and Nancy Cawley Pence, owned a chain of gas stations and convenience stores. After graduating from Columbus North High School in 1977, Pence attended Hanover College, a private liberal arts school affiliated with the Presbyterian Church. During his college years, he broke away from his Roman Catholic upbringing to become a born-again Christian. Although Pence had volunteered for Democratic candidates during high school, his political views also grew more conservative around this time.

After receiving a bachelor's degree in history from Hanover in 1981, Pence went on to earn a law degree from Indiana University in 1986. During his time in law school, he met and married his wife, Karen, an educator and artist. They eventually had three children, Michael, Charlotte, and Audrey. Pence spent the next few years working as an attorney and attempting to launch a political career. Running as a Republican, he unsuccessfully challenged Democratic incumbent Philip Sharp for his seat in the U.S. House of Representatives in 1988 and 1990. Over the next decade, Pence established his political credentials and raised his public profile by hosting public affairs radio and television programs. He started out by hosting a weekly half-hour radio show called *Washington Update with Mike Pence* on WRCR-FM in Rushville, Indiana. In 1992, Pence began offering conservative political commentary on his own daily program, *The Mike Pence Show,* which was eventually syndicated to 18 radio stations statewide. In 1995, Pence became host of a weekly television talk show on WNDY in Indianapolis. He also served as president of the Indiana Policy Review Foundation, a think tank devoted to free-market policy ideas.

In 2000, Pence mounted a successful campaign to represent Indiana's second congressional district in the U.S. House of Representatives. He went on to win reelection five times, representing the renumbered sixth congressional district from 2002 through 2013. Often describing himself as "a Christian, a conservative, and a Republican—in that order" (Garcia 2016), Pence quickly gained a reputation as one of the most conservative members of Congress and a vocal proponent of traditional family values, limited government, low taxes, fiscal responsibility, and strict adherence to the U.S. Constitution. In 2009, his colleagues unanimously elected him chairman of the House Republican Conference.

In 2012, Pence decided to run for governor of Indiana when the Republican incumbent, Mitch Daniels, stepped down due to term limits. Pence narrowly defeated Democrat John R. Gregg and took office as the state's 50th governor in January 2013. During his tenure, Pence enacted a major tax cut and invested more than $800 million in infrastructure projects. He also oversaw a job creation initiative that cut the state's unemployment rate in half. In addition, Pence established a state-funded Pre-K plan, expanded school choice programs, and emphasized career and technical education in high schools. As a conservative Christian, Pence signed several bills intended to restrict abortion rights in Indiana. In 2015, he also signed the Religious Freedom Restoration Act, which ostensibly prohibited the government from interfering with the free exercise of religion by individuals, businesses, or organizations. Opponents of the bill viewed it as a response to the nationwide legalization of same-sex marriage and claimed it would permit discrimination against LGBTQ people in the guise of "religious freedom." The intense backlash—including threatened boycotts of the state by major organizations—convinced Pence to sign a clarifying amendment that protected the rights of LGBTQ people.

Pence also faced controversy over his handling of an outbreak of human immunodeficiency virus (HIV)—the virus that causes acquired immune deficiency syndrome (AIDS)—in southern Indiana in late 2014 and early 2015. Some critics associated the outbreak with the governor's successful efforts to defund Planned Parenthood in the state, which led to the closure of several rural health clinics that offered AIDS prevention programs and HIV testing services. Pence also opposed publicly funded needle exchange programs, despite scientific evidence showing that they reduced the spread of disease by giving intravenous drug users access to sterile syringes. Once the HIV outbreak began, Pence refused to lift a state ban on funding for needle exchange programs, citing moral concerns that such programs encouraged substance abuse. Although Indiana eventually put the programs in place, critics charged that the governor's delayed response contributed to a worsening of the epidemic.

In 2016, Pence suspended his campaign for reelection as governor of Indiana to accept the Republican Party's nomination for vice president of the United States on a ticket headed by Donald Trump, a wealthy businessman and television personality. Political observers noted that the two running mates appeared to be opposites in terms of temperament, character, and experience. Pence's calm, self-effacing manner, moral rectitude, and resume as a governor and six-term member of Congress provided a stark contrast with Trump's bombastic style, playboy reputation, and outsider status. Analysts predicted that the addition of Pence would increase the ticket's appeal among evangelical Christians, political conservatives, and swing-state voters in the Midwest. Although some of Trump's statements and behavior posed a challenge to Pence's religious convictions—such as the release of the *Access Hollywood* tape, which recorded the nominee using crude language to boast that his celebrity entitled him to grope women—Pence remained a steadfast supporter throughout the campaign. "He has been seen as Trump's Christian conservative moral compass," Vox writer Tara Golshan (2017) explained, "there to assure the evangelical base that the Trump agenda would be in line with the values of the religious right."

After Trump prevailed over Democratic candidate Hillary Clinton in the 2016 election, Pence took office as the 48th vice president of the United States in January 2017. He served as chairman of the new administration's transition team and played an influential role in selecting Trump's cabinet. Only three weeks after taking office, Pence used his position as president of the Senate to cast the tie-breaking vote to confirm Betsy DeVos as Secretary of Education. He went on to break a dozen more ties during his first term in office—more than any other vice president in the modern era—including one that occurred during the debate over the Tax Cuts and Jobs Act of 2017, the passage of which ranked among Trump's signature legislative achievements. Pence also worked with Republican leaders in Congress to achieve the president's policy goals, and he represented the administration on several high-profile overseas trips to visit with foreign dignitaries and negotiate trade deals.

Although the Trump administration experienced an unusually high rate of turnover among top officials—often because individuals fell out of favor with the president—Pence remained in good standing by being loyal, dependable, and deferential. He frequently praised Trump's performance and never disagreed publicly with the administration's policies, even when they generated controversy. Historian Joel K. Goldstein, an expert in the constitutional role of the vice president, dubbed Pence the "sycophant-in-chief" and argued that his "obsequious" and "servile" behavior eroded the function of his office (Goldstein 2020). Yet other observers claimed that Pence wielded significant influence behind the scenes—operating as a "shadow president" (D'Antonio and Eisner 2018)—while also distancing himself from Trump's more outrageous statements and less popular policies. "The cumulative effect of Mr. Pence's conduct is to create around him a kind of artificial bubble of relative normalcy, in which the vice president avoids Mr. Trump's most explosive and divisive behavior mostly by pretending it does not exist," according to Alexander Burns and Maggie Haberman of the *New York Times* (2020).

The Trump administration faced its greatest challenge in early 2020, when a novel coronavirus emerged in China and quickly spread to other countries. In many people who became infected, the SARS-CoV-2 virus caused a severe and sometimes fatal respiratory illness called COVID-19. The first confirmed U.S. case of COVID-19 appeared in Washington State on January 20. Nine days later, Trump established the White House Coronavirus Task Force under the leadership of Secretary of Health and Human Services Alex Azar and assigned it a mission to "monitor, contain, and mitigate the spread of the virus, while ensuring that the American people have the most accurate and up-to-date health and travel information" (Santucci 2020).

On February 26, Trump announced that Pence would replace Azar as chair of the coronavirus task force. "The president wanted to make it clear to the American people that we're going to bring a whole of government approach to this," Pence explained (Santucci 2020). Some observers praised the move, claiming that it reflected the administration's growing prioritization of the COVID-19 crisis. Yet critics questioned the vice president's qualifications to coordinate the national response to a public health emergency, citing his lack of medical background and the disregard for scientific evidence he had shown when faced with an HIV epidemic as governor of Indiana. Some political analysts speculated that Trump elevated Pence to the highly visible role in order to have a scapegoat if the United States failed to contain the virus.

Upon taking over as chair, Pence expanded the task force to include more than a dozen new members, including Deborah Birx, a respected immunologist and AIDS researcher. He also earned praise for his calm, direct approach in conducting the group's daily press briefings. Pence provided statistical updates and answered reporters' questions about the federal response, but he deferred to medical professionals for detailed explanations of transmission methods, treatment approaches, and vaccine development. The tenor of the briefings changed dramatically on March 16, when Trump began conducting them himself. Rather than focusing on the COVID-19 pandemic, according to critics, Trump often used the platform to praise his administration's performance, attack his political opponents, engage in verbal sparring with reporters, and tout signs of a quick economic recovery. In addition, Trump frequently downplayed the severity of the virus and provided misinformation that contradicted medical experts. "The president loves to hype whatever he's offering, in this case the message that everything is fine," said Pence biographer Michael D'Antonio. "Pence has done a better job than I expected of honoring the science" (Smith 2020).

Pence's duties as task force chair also included coordinating federal assistance to states dealing with coronavirus outbreaks. As a former governor, the vice president received praise for his attentiveness to state concerns and his diplomacy in working with governors from both political parties during a series of weekly video conference calls. While Trump publicly rebuked governors who complained about shortages of testing materials, protective equipment, or ventilators, Pence worked behind the scenes to help them address the issues. Pence also came under criticism, however, for some elements of the administration's coronavirus response. Like the president, he sometimes resisted public health recommendations to wear a face mask and observe social-distancing guidelines. In April, for instance, Pence was photographed without a mask—in violation of hospital rules—during a visit to the Mayo Clinic in Minnesota. The vice president also echoed some of Trump's false or misleading claims about the virus. When the nation experienced a second wave of COVID-19 cases in June, for example, Pence attributed the surge to an expansion of testing capacity. Since the percentage of positive tests grew as well as the number of tests conducted, public health experts blamed the rise in COVID-19 cases on the relaxation of stay-at-home orders.

Despite some early rumors that Trump might replace Pence on the ticket for his 2020 reelection bid, Pence's loyalty earned him the vice presidential nomination once again. In his acceptance speech at the

Republican National Convention, Pence praised the administration's coronavirus response—describing it as "the greatest national mobilization since World War II"—and proclaimed the crisis to be nearly over. "America is a nation of miracles and we're on track to have the world's first safe, effective coronavirus vaccine by the end of this year," he stated. "After all the sacrifice in this year like no other—all the hardship—we are finding our way forward again" (Cassidy 2020). Pointing out that COVID-19 had claimed 180,000 American lives and showed few signs of abating, *New Yorker* columnist John Cassidy (2020) called Pence's speech "the ultimate rewriting of history" and "a travesty of the truth."

Further Reading

Burns, Alexander, and Maggie Haberman. 2020. "From Trump's Shadow, Mike Pence Can See 2024." *New York Times,* August 26, 2020. https://www.nytimes.com/2020/08/26/us/politics/mike-pence-trump-vp.html.

Cassidy, John. 2020. "Mike Pence's Big Lie about Trump and the Coronavirus at the Republican National Convention." *New Yorker,* August 27, 2020. https://www.newyorker.com/news/our-columnists/mike-pences-big-lie-about-trump-and-the-coronavirus-at-the-republican-national-convention.

D'Antonio, Michael, and Peter Eisner. 2018. *The Shadow President: The Truth about Mike Pence.* New York: St. Martin's.

Garcia, Catherine. 2016. "Mike Pence: 'I'm a Christian, a Conservative, and a Republican—in That Order." *The Week,* July 20, 2016. https://theweek.com/speedreads/637487/mike-pence-im-christian-conservative-republican—that-order.

Goldstein, Joel K. 2020. "Trump Has Made Pence the Sycophant-in-Chief. That's Why He's Keeping Him." NBC News, August 23, 2020. https://www.nbcnews.com/think/opinion/trump-has-made-mike-pence-sycophant-chief-s-why-he-ncna1045436.

Golshan, Tara. 2017. "Mike Pence's Tie-Breaking Vote Was Key to Republicans' Strategy in 2017." Vox, December 29, 2017. https://www.vox.com/2017/12/29/16821628/mike-pence-tie-break-republicans-2017.

LoBianco, Tom. 2019. *Piety and Power: Mike Pence and the Taking of the White House.* New York: HarperCollins.

Santucci, Jeanine. 2020. "What We Know about the Coronavirus Task Force Now That Mike Pence Is in Charge." *USA Today,* February 27, 2020. https://www.usatoday.com/story/news/politics/2020/02/27/coronavirus-what-we-know-mike-pence-and-task-force/4891905002/.

Smith, David. 2020. "Strangely Competent Mike Pence Finds His 9/11 Moment in Coronavirus Crisis." *Guardian,* March 21, 2020. https://www.theguardian.com/us-news/2020/mar/21/mike-pence-coronavirus-crisis.

Donald Trump (1946–)

President of the United States during the COVID-19 pandemic

Donald John Trump was born on June 14, 1946, in the Queens borough of New York City. His father, Frederick Trump, was a wealthy real estate developer, and his mother, Mary Anne MacLeod Trump, was a homemaker. As the fourth of five children in his family, Trump enjoyed a privileged childhood in the Jamaica Estates neighborhood of Queens. He completed his early education at the private Kew-Forest School before attending boarding school at the New York Military Academy, where he played golf and football. After graduating in 1964, Trump spent two years at Fordham University before transferring to the Wharton School of Business at the University of Pennsylvania. Trump received several draft deferments to avoid military service during the Vietnam War, including student deferments during his college years and medical deferments that he claimed were due to bone spurs in his feet.

After earning a bachelor's degree in economics from Wharton in 1968, Trump went to work for his father's real estate development company, E. Trump and Son. Three years later, Trump became president of the company and renamed it The Trump Organization. Under his leadership, the company shifted its development emphasis from middle-class rental housing to luxury hotels, casinos, resorts, and golf courses. In 1980, Trump launched the construction of Trump Tower, a 58-story Manhattan skyscraper that served as the headquarters of his business empire as well as his personal residence. In 1985, he purchased Mar-a-Lago, a private, luxury estate in Palm Beach, Florida. Trump eventually expanded his business interests to include a variety of other ventures. He operated an airline, for instance, served as a promoter for professional boxing and wrestling matches, launched a real estate training program called Trump University, and produced the Miss Universe beauty pageant. In 1987, Trump published a best-selling book outlining his business philosophy, *The Art of the Deal*.

Trump also established himself as a television personality. Beginning in 2003, he spent 14 seasons as producer and host of *The Apprentice*, a reality competition show that originally aired on NBC. On each episode, teams of contestants completed business-related tasks as Trump and expert advisers looked on and evaluated their performance. Afterward, Trump selected one contestant to eliminate from the competition with the catchphrase, "You're fired!" The final contestant remaining at the end of the season-long competition won a $250,000 job in The Trump Organization.

As Trump's celebrity grew, he also made cameo and guest appearances on many television series and radio programs.

Over the years, Trump occasionally discussed political ambitions that included serving as president of the United States. He formed an exploratory committee to consider running for president in 2000 as a Reform Party candidate, for instance, before becoming a member of the Democratic Party in 2001. Eight years later, following the election of Democrat Barack Obama as the 44th president, Trump switched his allegiance to the Republican Party. He emerged as an outspoken critic of the Obama administration's policies, as well as a prominent "birther" who promoted the false conspiracy theory that Obama was born in Africa and thus did not meet the constitutional citizenship requirements to be president. Trump's status among Republicans rose following his keynote addresses to party leaders at the Conservative Political Action Conference (CPAC) in 2011 and 2013.

In 2015, Trump launched a formal bid for the Republican nomination for president. As the least experienced among 17 candidates in the primaries, he did not get much respect from political analysts, but his brash personality and bold proposals received significant media attention. Trump also gathered populist support with his raucous campaign rallies and promise to "Make America Great Again." After capturing the Republican nomination, he faced off against Democratic nominee Hillary Clinton, the former secretary of state, U.S. senator, and first lady, in the 2016 election. During his campaign, Trump vowed to build a wall along the 1,900-mile Mexican border to prevent immigrants from entering the country illegally. He also promised to repeal the Affordable Care Act and dismantle climate change regulations that Obama had put in place. Finally, Trump pledged to create a pro-business climate by lowering taxes, reducing regulations, and renegotiating unfair trade agreements.

Trump came under criticism throughout his presidential campaign for making false or misleading statements. When the mainstream press questioned his assertions, Trump claimed to be the victim of biased media coverage and "fake news." Critics also uncovered evidence suggesting that Trump engaged in shady business deals, exaggerated his wealth, and paid "hush money" to bury negative information. Shortly before the November election, Trump became embroiled in scandal over a leaked tape in which he made sexually explicit comments and appeared to suggest that his fame entitled him to grope women. Trump also made several remarks during his campaign that critics condemned as racist, such as when he characterized Mexican immigrants as criminals, drug dealers, and rapists.

Although Clinton held a commanding lead in polls leading up to the election and won the popular vote, Trump prevailed in the Electoral College and claimed the presidency. He thus became the first person to be elected president without previous government or military service. Most political analysts considered his victory a shocking upset. Surveys showed that he garnered strong support among conservative, rural white voters driven by racial resentment and economic insecurity. In addition, investigations by U.S. security agencies found evidence of Russian interference in the election aimed at helping Trump, particularly through fake social media posts intended to inflame partisan debate and foment public discord. A progressive resistance movement formed to oppose Trump's presidency, and followers organized several large-scale protests as he prepared to take office. Millions of people around the world participated in the Women's March, for instance, on the day following Trump's inauguration.

As president, Trump followed through on his promise to restrict legal immigration and crack down on unauthorized border crossing. Although he failed to convince Congress to provide funding to build a wall, Trump enacted a controversial deterrent policy in 2018 that resulted in thousands of Central American migrant children being separated from their families at the U.S.-Mexico border. He rescinded the policy following a public outcry, and immigration agencies reunified most of the migrant families under a federal court order. Trump also aroused controversy by expressing support for white supremacist and neo-Nazi demonstrators involved in a violent clash with counter protesters over the removal of a Confederate statue in Charlottesville, Virginia, in 2017. Critics interpreted the president's statement that there were "fine people on both sides" of the conflict as implying moral equivalency between racist and anti-racist positions (Haltiwanger 2019).

One of Trump's signature achievements came with the passage of the Tax Cuts and Jobs Act of 2017, which made major revisions to the federal tax code. Proponents asserted that the law would create jobs and promote economic growth, but critics claimed that the changes favored wealthy Americans and large corporations. Trump also reshaped the U.S. judiciary by appointing three conservative Supreme Court justices and more than 200 conservative federal judges to lifetime terms on the bench. In addition, Trump withdrew the United States from the Paris Climate Agreement and renegotiated several international trade agreements, arguing that these deals disadvantaged American business interests. Although Trump presided over a strong U.S. economy and soaring stock market values, critics pointed out that the upward trajectory had started before he took office.

The Trump administration faced its greatest challenge in early 2020, when a novel coronavirus emerged in China and quickly spread to other countries. In many people who became infected, the SARS-CoV-2 virus caused a severe and sometimes fatal respiratory illness called COVID-19.

The first confirmed U.S. case of COVID-19 appeared in Washington State on January 20 in a man who had recently traveled to China. The next day, Trump insisted that he was not worried about a major outbreak occurring in the United States. "We have it totally under control," he declared. "It's one person coming in from China, and we have it under control. It's going to be just fine" (Leonhardt 2020). According to critics, this response marked the beginning of a seven-week period in which Trump ignored warnings from medical experts, downplayed the severity of COVID-19, promoted conspiracy theories and fake cures, and failed to prepare the nation for the impending public health crisis. Yale University physician and sociologist Nicholas Christakis said administration officials could have used this time "to build ventilators, get protective equipment, organize our ICUs, get tests ready, prepare the public for what was going to happen so that our economy didn't tank as badly. None of this was done adequately by our leaders" (Fallows 2020).

On January 31, Trump suspended travel to the United States from China. He often mentioned this action as an example of his aggressive response to the coronavirus. Since the restrictions only applied to foreign nationals and not to American citizens or their immediate family members, however, an estimated 40,000 people still entered the country from China after they took effect. For most of February, as cases increased in Asia and Europe, Trump minimized the threat posed by COVID-19. For instance, he falsely claimed the disease was no worse than the seasonal flu, asserted without evidence that the coronavirus would disappear with the arrival of warmer weather, and described warnings of an approaching pandemic as a Democratic "hoax" intended to cause a public panic, sink the U.S. economy, and harm his reelection campaign.

Countries that successfully halted the spread of the coronavirus implemented extensive testing protocols to identify and isolate carriers—some of whom never developed symptoms—and deploy personnel and resources to contain outbreaks. In the United States, however, coronavirus testing became mired in problems, delays, and political wrangling. On March 6, Trump (2020) declared that "anybody that needs a test gets a test." In reality, supply shortages and logistical issues limited the availability of tests, forcing public health officials to reserve them for symptomatic patients with known exposure or a history of travel to affected areas. Meanwhile, Trump touted the relatively low number of COVID-19 cases in the United States compared to other countries, even as public health officials warned that the lack of testing allowed the virus to spread undetected.

On March 16, Trump began appearing at the daily, televised press briefings held by the White House Coronavirus Task Force—a panel he had convened six weeks earlier to provide the American people with up-to-date information about COVID-19. After the president downplayed the severity of the crisis for nearly two months, some observers viewed his participation as evidence of a shift toward acknowledging the urgency of the situation and promoting measures intended to contain the spread of the virus. In the eyes of critics, however, Trump's appearances in the task force briefings did little to inform or reassure the public. Rather than focusing on the COVID-19 pandemic, Trump often used the platform to praise his administration's performance, attack his political opponents, engage in verbal sparring with reporters, and tout signs of a quick economic recovery. In addition, Trump frequently provided misinformation that contradicted medical experts. He repeatedly touted the antimalaria drug hydroxychloroquine as a potential cure before it had been tested, for instance, and he once made the dangerous suggestion that COVID-19 patients consume or inject disinfectants. Trump also refused to wear a face mask in accordance with public health recommendations, which encouraged some of his followers to eschew mask wearing as a political statement.

In the absence of a coordinated national strategy, state governors implemented their own measures to combat the spread of the coronavirus. California became the first state to issue a stay-at-home order on March 19, and most other states enacted similar restrictions over the next week. Some governors expressed frustration with Trump and criticized what they viewed as a lack of federal leadership and support. Trump responded by claiming that the states had everything they should need, blaming the governors for mishandling the crisis, and dismissing the complaints as politically motivated. Tensions rose in April as the virtual shutdown in the operations of most states caused mass unemployment and economic hardship nationwide. Trump increasingly asserted his authority and pressured governors to lift restrictions and reopen their states. Some critics charged that the mixed messages coming from state and federal authorities caused confusion, weakened citizens' commitment to following social-distancing measures, and contributed to a resurgence of COVID-19 cases in June and July.

On March 27, Trump signed the Coronavirus Aid, Relief, and Economic Security (CARES) Act into law. At $2.2 trillion, it marked the largest stimulus package ever passed in U.S. history. The CARES Act provided one-time economic impact payments to more than 150 million Americans, temporarily boosted unemployment compensation, and provided loans and other aid to help small businesses, large corporations, and state and local governments weather the crisis. Nevertheless, the coronavirus remained a threat and continued to disrupt Americans' daily lives throughout the summer of 2020. An August poll conducted by the Kaiser Family Foundation found that 61 percent of voters disapproved of Trump's handling of the pandemic, while only 35 percent approved (Kirzinger, Kearney, and Hamel 2020). By November, the United States had recorded 10 million cases of COVID-19—around one-fifth of the world total—and nearly 250,000 deaths. Public dissatisfaction with the administration's coronavirus response contributed to Trump's defeat in the presidential election.

In his personal life, Trump has been married three times—to Czech model Ivana Zelníčková (1977–1992), actress Marla Maples (1993–1999), and Slovenian model Melania Knauss (2005–)—and has five children, Donald Jr., Ivanka, Eric, Tiffany, and Barron.

Further Reading

"Donald Trump Fast Facts." CNN, September 4, 2019. https://www.cnn.com /2013/07/04/us/donald-trump-fast-facts/index.html.

Fallows, James. 2020. "The Three Weeks That Changed Everything." *Atlantic,* June 29, 2020. https://www.theatlantic.com/politics/archive/2020/06/how -white-house-coronavirus-response-went-wrong/613591/.

Haltiwanger, John. 2019. "Trump's Biggest Accomplishments and Failures as President as He Heads into an Election Year after Impeachment." *Business Insider,* December 31, 2019. https://www.businessinsider.com/trump -biggest-accomplishments-and-failures-heading-into-2020-2019-12.

Kirzinger, Ashley, Audrey Kearney, and Liz Hamel. 2020. "Voters Are Souring on President Trump's Handling of the Coronavirus, with Implications for November." Kaiser Family Foundation, August 17, 2020. https://www.kff .org/policy-watch/voters-are-souring-on-president-trumps-handling-of -coronavirus-with-implications-for-november/.

Leonhardt, David. 2020. "A Complete List of Trump's Attempts to Play Down Coronavirus." *New York Times,* March 15, 2020. https://www.nytimes .com/2020/03/15/opinion/trump-coronavirus.html.

Peters, Cameron. 2020. "A Detailed Timeline of All the Ways Trump Failed to Respond to the Coronavirus." Vox, June 8, 2020. https://www.vox.com /2020/6/8/21242003/trump-failed-coronavirus-response.

"President Trump's Historic Coronavirus Response." The White House, August 10, 2020. https://www.whitehouse.gov/briefings-statements/president-trumps -historic-coronavirus-response/.

Trump, Donald. 2020. "Remarks by President Trump after Tour of the Centers for Disease Control and Prevention, Atlanta, Georgia." The White House, March 7, 2020. https://www.whitehouse.gov/briefings-statements/remarks -president-trump-tour-centers-disease-control-prevention-atlanta-ga/.

Gretchen Whitmer (1971–)

Governor of Michigan during the COVID-19 pandemic

Gretchen Esther Whitmer was born on August 23, 1971, in Lansing, the state capital of Michigan. Both of her parents were attorneys who held influential positions in the state government. Her father, Richard, led the state Department of Commerce under Republican Governor William Milliken (served 1969–1983) and later became president and CEO of Blue Cross Blue Shield of Michigan. Her mother, Sherry, worked as an assistant attorney general under Democratic Attorney General Frank J. Kelley (served 1961–1999). Whitmer and her two younger siblings, Liz and Richard Jr., grew up in a nonpartisan household with a deep commitment to public service. "Neither one of them were ideologues," Whitmer recalled of her parents. "My mom probably would have been described like a Reagan Democrat, and my dad was a Milliken Republican. In Michigan, that's theoretically a Democrat and a Republican, but it's pretty close on the scale" (Alberta 2020).

When Whitmer was ten years old, her parents divorced and the children moved with their mother to Grand Rapids, an hour west of Lansing. After graduating from Forest Hills Central High School near Grand Rapids in 1989, Whitmer went on to attend Michigan State University (MSU) in East Lansing. Through most of her college years, Whitmer planned to become a sportscaster, and she interned in the MSU athletic department. After her junior year, however, her father convinced her to broaden her perspective by spending a semester working at the state capitol. He arranged an internship in the office of Curtis Hertel, a powerful Democrat who represented Detroit in Michigan's House of Representatives for 18 years. The experience helped awaken Whitmer's political convictions. "From there on, I realized that I was a Democrat," she recalled (Alberta 2020).

Shifting her sights toward a career in politics, Whitmer started out by mounting a successful campaign for president of her sorority, Kappa Alpha Theta. After receiving a bachelor's degree in communications in 1993, Whitmer went on to attend law school at MSU, completing her law degree in 1998. She worked as an attorney in Lansing and volunteered for local Democratic candidates until a House seat opened up in 2000. At the age of twenty-eight, Whitmer decided to run for office. "It was less about politics and party and more about civic responsibility," said her sister, Liz Gereghty. "[Our parents] gave us this sense that there should be meaning in your lives. There should be some good that you're doing in the world. Some jobs are more important than others" (Heller 2020). The political newcomer used her family connections to raise three times as much money as any other candidate in the race. After squeaking out a 281-vote victory in the hotly contested Democratic primary, Whitmer cruised to victory in the general election.

Whitmer's first two-year term coincided with a series of challenges in her personal life, as she gave birth to her first child and also took care of her mother, who was diagnosed with a lethal form of brain cancer. "They say that the five most stressful life events are getting married, having a child, the death of a loved one, moving your house, and starting a new job. And I did all of those things in that same two-year period," she remembered (Alberta 2020). "The way that I got through that period of time was not thinking about the 100 yards down the road but looking at the next five [yards] . . . and staying optimistic" (Heller 2020). Nevertheless, the freshman legislator managed to impress her colleagues on both sides of the aisle. "We could tell right away she was an up-and-comer," said former Republican state representative Randy Richardville. "She just had a presence about her. She's a very intelligent woman. She wasn't trying to stand out in those days, but she's got some natural skills and abilities that were easy to notice" (Alberta 2020).

Whitmer won reelection to the House in 2002 and 2004. In 2006, she was elected to the first of two four-year terms in the Michigan Senate. Although she was badly outnumbered as both a woman and a Democrat, Whitmer earned a reputation as a pragmatist able to forge agreements on legislation. "I think of myself as someone who is progressive but also can get stuff done. And I don't vilify people that don't see the world precisely the same way I do," she stated. "Fourteen years in the minority keeps you humble and helps you focus on opportunities to seize on when you know you can make a difference" (Alberta 2020). In 2011, Whitmer's fellow Democrats unanimously chose her as the first female leader of a party caucus in the state senate. In this role, she often marshaled opposition to the policies of Republican Governor Rick Snyder (served 2011–2019).

In 2013, Whitmer made national headlines for an impassioned floor speech she made during the debate over a proposed bill that would require Michigan women to purchase special insurance to cover abortion, even in cases of rape or incest. She sent shockwaves through the chamber by revealing that she had been a victim of rape while in college. "Thank God it didn't result in a pregnancy, because I can't imagine going through what I went through then have to consider what to do about an unwanted pregnancy from an attacker," Whitmer said. "If this were law then, and I had become pregnant, I would not have been able to have coverage because of this. . . . I'm not enjoying talking about it. It's something I've hidden for a long time. But I think you need to see the face of the women you are impacting by this vote today" (Alberta 2020). Although her speech did not prevent the bill from passing, Whitmer felt gratified that it empowered hundreds of sexual assault victims from across the country to tell their own stories.

In 2015, Whitmer left office due to term limits and briefly returned to private life. The following year, she served as Ingham County prosecutor for six months after the incumbent resigned due to his involvement in a prostitution scandal. In 2017, Whitmer announced her intention to run for governor of Michigan to replace Snyder, who faced term limits. After winning all 83 counties in the Democratic primary, she defeated Republican Attorney General Bill Schuette by a ten-point margin in the general election and took office as the state's 49th governor in January 2019. During her first year, Whitmer focused much of her attention on trying to fulfill her campaign promise to "fix the damn roads"—a reference to Michigan's notorious potholes and neglected bridges and infrastructure. Her proposal to finance road repairs with a 45-cent-per-gallon gasoline tax, however, proved unpopular with voters and encountered staunch resistance from the Republican-controlled state legislature. Some of Whitmer's other policy priorities included increasing funding for public education, expanding access to health care, providing clean drinking water, and ending discrimination on the basis of sexual orientation and gender identity.

In February 2020, Whitmer appeared on the national stage to deliver the Democratic response to President Donald Trump's State of the Union Address. At the end of that month, the United States recorded its first death due to COVID-19, a severe respiratory illness caused by a novel coronavirus that originated in China and quickly spread around the world. Although the first confirmed cases of COVID-19 did not appear in Michigan until March 10—the day before the World Health Organization declared it a global pandemic—the state quickly emerged as a hot spot, with the infection rate increasing rapidly and sick patients overwhelming hospitals. Whitmer responded quickly to the public health crisis. On March 12, she announced the temporary closure of all schools in the state. Four days later, she issued an order restricting bars and restaurants to carryout service and prohibiting all social gatherings larger than 50 people. On March 24, Whitmer imposed a statewide stay-at-home order that closed all nonessential businesses, restricted discretionary travel, and required individuals to remain at home except to acquire food, access medical care, or exercise outdoors.

In early April, with Michigan behind only New York and New Jersey in COVID-19 cases and deaths, Whitmer pleaded for federal assistance to address shortages of testing supplies, ventilators, and personal protective equipment (PPE) for medical workers. She also expressed frustration with the Trump administration's response to the pandemic and urged the federal government to implement a national strategy rather than forcing states to develop their own separate—and often conflicting—approaches. Trump responded angrily to the criticism in a series of tweets, dismissing Whitmer as "the woman in Michigan" and "Gretchen 'Half' Whitmer." The president also insinuated that he would provide federal assistance only to governors who seemed "appreciative" (Alberta 2020).

Trump's tweets pushed Whitmer and her coronavirus response into the national spotlight. She received a flood of media attention, with interviews on television news programs and profiles in newspapers and magazines. Whitmer even became the subject of a parody sketch on *Saturday Night Live.* "I was thrown into the spotlight by being criticized or attacked by the president of the United States. I didn't ask for that. I didn't like it," she said. "I would hate for anyone in Michigan to not have the help they need because I'm not popular with the president" (Graham 2020). As the controversy raised her public profile, Whitmer reportedly came under consideration as a potential vice presidential running mate for 2020 Democratic nominee Joe Biden. She insisted that her main focus remained on guiding her state through the pandemic. "I want people to understand how devastating this has been for Michigan," she said. "I know some people criticize this [publicity], but the irony is if I wasn't doing it, I wouldn't be doing my job well" (Heller 2020).

Whitmer came into conflict with Trump again in April, when the president began pushing states to reopen their economies. Instead, on the advice of public health experts, Whitmer extended her stay-at-home order several times and only partially lifted it on June 1. Although the restrictions succeeded in slowing the spread of the coronavirus—and polls showed that 72 percent of Michigan voters approved of the governor's handling of the crisis—Trump and some Michigan Republicans argued that Whitmer overstepped her authority, encroached on individual liberties, and unnecessarily harmed businesses. "A lot of the orders have been vague and confusing, and sometimes even mistakes," said state senator Ed McBroom (Heller 2020). Critics grew particularly incensed over restrictions that temporarily prevented residents from traveling to vacation homes within the state, launching powerboats, shopping at nurseries and garden-supply stores, and visiting barbershops and hair salons. Republican state legislators filed a series of lawsuits that eventually succeeded in curtailing some of Whitmer's emergency powers.

In late April and early May, right-wing groups organized protests in Lansing to express their objections to Whitmer's stay-at-home order.

Many of the anti-lockdown protesters wore "Make America Great Again" hats or waved flags promoting Trump's reelection campaign. Some demonstrators, dressed as militia members and carrying assault weapons, forced their way into the state capitol building. A few carried signs with racist symbols, and one protester hung a female mannequin from a noose. Although Whitmer expressed support for the people's right to protest, she objected to the some of the images and tactics used. "We know that people are not all happy about having to take the stay-home posture," she stated. "But we have to listen to the public health experts, and displays like the one we saw in our state capitol are not representative of who we are in Michigan. There were swastikas and Confederate flags and nooses and people with assault rifles. That's a small group of people when you think that this is a state of almost 10 million people, the vast majority of whom are doing the right thing" (Graham 2020).

Trump tweeted messages of support for the anti-lockdown protesters, encouraging them to "LIBERATE MICHIGAN." He also demanded that Whitmer loosen restrictions and reopen the state economy. "The governor of Michigan should give a little, and put out the fire. These are very good people, but they are angry. They want their lives back again, safely! See them, talk to them, make a deal" (Graham 2020). Although Whitmer refused to allow the president or protesters to dictate the reopening schedule, she gradually modified or lifted most of her orders in June and July. She looked forward to ending the crisis and returning to normal state business. "It's like nothing we ever imagined," she acknowledged. "There's no experience you can draw on to get through this. It has taken over everything. It *is* everything. I mean, all I talked about for three years was 'Fix the Damn Roads.' And now all I talk about is PPE, and I didn't even know what it was" (Alberta 2020). In her personal life, Whitmer has two daughters—Sherry and Sydney—from her marriage to Gary Shrewsbury, which ended in divorce in 2008. In 2011, she married Marc Mallory, a dentist who has three sons from a previous marriage—Alex, Mason, and Winston. They live in Lansing, Michigan.

Further Reading

Alberta, Tim. 2020. "'The Woman in Michigan' Goes National." Politico, April 9, 2020. https://www.politico.com/news/magazine/2020/04/09/gretchen -whitmer-governor-michigan-profile-2020-coronavirus-biden-vp-177791.

Graham, Bryan Arman. 2020. "'Swastikas and Nooses': Governor Slams 'Racism' of Michigan Lockdown Protest." *Guardian,* May 3, 2020. https://www.the guardian.com/us-news/2020/may/03/michigan-gretchen-whitmer-lock down-protest-racism.

Heller, Karen. 2020. "The Turbulent Rise of Gretchen Whitmer." *Washington Post,*
        June 2, 2020. https://www.washingtonpost.com/lifestyle/style/gretchen
        -whitmer-michigan-governor-trump-coronavirus/2020/06/01/98e8b108
        -9b6f-11ea-ac72-3841fcc9b35f_story.html.
Perkins, Tom. 2020. "'Big Gretch': How the Pandemic Pushed Michigan's Gover-
        nor into the Spotlight." *Guardian,* May 13, 2020. https://www.theguardian
        .com/us-news/2020/may/13/gretchen-whitmer-michigan-governor
        -coronavirus.
Shesgreen, Deirdre, and Maureen Groppe. 2020. "Anti-Quarantine Protests,
        Trump Pressure Put Governors on Political Tightrope over Coronavirus."
        USA Today, April 22, 2020. https://www.usatoday.com/story/news/world
        /2020/04/22/coronavirus-governors-michigan-whitmer-florida-desantis
        -key-states-face-trump-pressure-amid-response/5169260002/.
Soicher, Spencer. 2020. "President Trump and Governor Whitmer Exchange
        More Jabs." WILX, March 27, 2020. https://www.wilx.com/content/news
        /President-Trump-and-Gov-Whitmer-569155591.html.

Further Resources

Pandemic Preparedness

Akpan, Nsikan. 2020. "New Coronavirus Can Spread between Humans, but It Started in a Wildlife Market." *National Geographic,* January 21, 2020. https://www.nationalgeographic.com/science/2020/01/new-coronavirus -spreading-between-humans-how-it-started/.

Belluz, Julia. 2020. "Did China Downplay the Coronavirus Outbreak Early On?" Vox, January 27, 2020. https://www.vox.com/2020/1/27/21082354 /coronavirus-outbreak-wuhan-china-early-on-lancet.

Borio, Luciana, and Scott Gottlieb. 2020. "Act Now to Prevent an American Epidemic." *Wall Street Journal,* January 28, 2020. https://www.wsj.com /articles/act-now-to-prevent-an-american-epidemic-11580255335.

Brennan, Margaret, and Camilla Schick. 2020. "Finding Coronavirus' Patient Zero; and a Guilty Bat." CBS News, May 7, 2020. https://www.cbsnews .com/news/coronavirus-patient-zero-bat-index-case/.

Christakis, Nicholas A. 2020. *Apollo's Arrow: The Profound and Enduring Impact of Coronavirus on the Way We Live.* New York: Hachette.

Crossley, Gabriel. 2020. "Wuhan Lockdown 'Unprecedented,' Shows Commitment to Contain Virus: Who Representative in China." Reuters, January 23, 2020. https://www.reuters.com/article/us-china-health-who-idU SKBN1ZM1G9.

Cyranoski, David. 2020. "What China's Coronavirus Response Can Teach the Rest of the World." *Nature,* March 17, 2020. https://www.nature.com /articles/d41586-020-00741-x.

Diamond, Dan. 2020. "Inside America's Two-Decade Failure to Prepare for Coronavirus." Politico, April 11, 2020. https://www.politico.com/news/magazine /2020/04/11/america-two-decade-failure-prepare-coronavirus-179574.

Ducharme, Jamie. 2020. "World Health Organization Declares COVID-19 a 'Pandemic.' Here's What That Means." *Time,* March 11, 2020. https://time .com/5791661/who-coronavirus-pandemic-declaration/.

Editorial Board. 2020. "Here Comes the Coronavirus Pandemic." *New York Times,* February 29, 2020. https://www.nytimes.com/2020/02/29/opinion/sunday/corona-virus-usa.html.

Fidler, David P. 2020. "Coronavirus: A Twenty-Year Failure." Think Global Health, March 23, 2020. https://www.thinkglobalhealth.org/article/coronavirus-twenty-year-failure.

Kuo, Lily. 2020. "Coronavirus: Wuhan Doctor Speaks Out against Authorities." *Guardian,* March 11, 2020. https://www.theguardian.com/world/2020/mar/11/coronavirus-wuhan-doctor-ai-fen-speaks-out-against-authorities.

Lakoff, Andrew. 2017. *Unprepared: Global Health in the Time of Emergency.* Berkeley: University of California Press.

LePan, Nicholas. 2020. "Ranked: Global Pandemic Preparedness by Country." Visual Capitalist, March 20, 2020. https://www.visualcapitalist.com/global-pandemic-preparedness-ranked/.

Letzter, Rafi. 2020. "The Coronavirus Didn't Really Start at That Wuhan 'Wet Market.'" LiveScience, May 28, 2020. https://www.livescience.com/covid-19-did-not-start-at-wuhan-wet-market.html.

Lewis, Wayne. 2020. "Disaster Response Expert Explains Why U.S. Wasn't More Prepared for the Pandemic." USC Dornsife, March 24, 2020. https://dornsife.usc.edu/news/stories/3182/why-u-s-wasnt-better-prepared-for-the-coronavirus/.

Ma, Josephine. 2020. "Coronavirus: China's First COVID-19 Case Traced Back to November 17." *South China Morning Post,* March 13, 2020. https://www.scmp.com/news/china/society/article/3074991/coronavirus-chinas-first-confirmed-covid-19-case-traced-back.

Mackenzie, J. S., P. Drury, A. Ellis, T. Grein, K. C. Leitmeyer, S. Mardel, A. Merianos, B. Olowokure, C. Roth, R. Slattery, G. Thomson, D. Werker, and M. Ryan. 2004. "The WHO Response to SARS and Preparations for the Future." In *Learning from SARS: Preparing for the Next Disease Outbreak*, edited by Stacey Knobler, Adel Mahmoud, Stanley Lemon, Alison Mack, Laura Sivitz, and Katherine Oberholtzer. Washington, DC: National Academies Press, 2004. https://www.ncbi.nlm.nih.gov/books/NBK92476/.

Madrigal, Alexis C., and Robinson Meyer. 2020. "How the Coronavirus Became an American Catastrophe." *Atlantic,* March 21, 2020. https://www.theatlantic.com/health/archive/2020/03/how-many-americans-are-sick-lost-february/608521/.

Pisano, Gary P., Raffaella Sadun, and Michele Zanini. 2020. "Lessons from Italy's Response to Coronavirus." *Harvard Business Review,* March 27, 2020. https://hbr.org/2020/03/lessons-from-italys-response-to-coronavirus.

Radcliffe, Shawn. 2020. "Can We Learn Anything from the SARS Outbreak to Fight COVID-19?" Healthline, March 11, 2020. https://www.healthline.com/health-news/has-anything-changed-since-the-2003-sars-outbreak.

Rieder, Rem. 2020. "Contrary to Trump's Claim, a Pandemic Was Widely Expected at Some Point." FactCheck.org, March 20, 2020. https://www.factcheck.org/2020/03/contrary-to-trumps-claim-a-pandemic-was-widely-expected-at-some-point/.

Taylor, Derrick Bryson. 2020. "A Timeline of the Coronavirus Pandemic." *New York Times,* August 6, 2020. https://www.nytimes.com/article/coronavirus-timeline.html?auth=login-google.

Thompson, Derek. 2020. "What's Behind South Korea's COVID-19 Exceptionalism?" *Atlantic,* May 6, 2020. https://www.theatlantic.com/ideas/archive/2020/05/whats-south-koreas-secret/611215/.

Yu, Verna. 2020. "'Hero Who Told the Truth': Chinese Rage over Coronavirus Death of Whistleblower Doctor." *Guardian,* February 7, 2020. https://www.theguardian.com/global-development/2020/feb/07/coronavirus-chinese-rage-death-whistleblower-doctor-li-wenliang.

The Trump Administration's Response

Alexander, Erik B. 2020. "Beating COVID-19 Demands President Trump Work With, Not Against, Governors." *Washington Post,* April 13, 2020. https://www.washingtonpost.com/outlook/2020/04/03/beating-covid-19-demands-president-trump-work-with-not-against-governors/.

Altman, Drew. 2020. "Public Wants Federal Government, Not States, in Charge on Coronavirus." Axios, April 7, 2020. https://www.axios.com/states-federal-government-coronavirus-trump-b999862d-3e08-46f4-8707-d9d6ab213671.html.

Benen, Steve. 2020. "On Virus Missteps, Trump Declares, 'I Don't Take Responsibility at All.'" MSNBC, March 16, 2020. https://www.msnbc.com/rachel-maddow-show/virus-missteps-trump-declares-i-don-t-take-responsibility-all-n1160236.

Blake, Aaron. 2020. "Two Months in the Dark: The Increasingly Damning Timeline of Trump's Coronavirus Response." *Washington Post,* April 21, 2020. https://www.washingtonpost.com/politics/2020/04/07/timeline-trumps-coronavirus-response-is-increasingly-damning/.

Bump, Philip, and Ashley Parker. 2020. "13 Hours of Trump." *Washington Post,* April 26, 2020. https://www.washingtonpost.com/politics/13-hours-of-trump-the-president-fills-briefings-with-attacks-and-boasts-but-little-empathy/2020/04/25/7eec5ab0-8590-11ea-a3eb-e9fc93160703_story.html.

Capehart, Jonathan. 2020. "Susan Rice on Trump's Coronavirus Response: 'He Has Cost Thousands of American Lives.'" *Washington Post,* April 6, 2020. https://www.washingtonpost.com/opinions/2020/04/06/susan-rice-trumps-coronavirus-response-he-has-cost-tens-thousands-american-lives/.

Cathey, Libby. 2020. "Coronavirus Government Response Updates: Trump Signs $2T Relief Bill after House Passage." ABC News, March 27, 2020.

https://abcnews.go.com/Politics/coronavirus-government-response
-updates-drama-house-votes-2t/story?id=69833576.

Choi, Matthew. 2020. "Trump Calls Inslee a 'Snake' over Criticism of Coronavirus Rhetoric." Politico, March 6, 2020. https://www.politico.com/news
/2020/03/06/donald-trump-jay-inslee-coronavirus-123114.

Eder, Steve, Henry Fountain, Michael H. Keller, Muyi Xiao, and Alexandra Stevenson. 2020. "430,000 People Have Traveled from China to U.S. since Coronavirus Surfaced." *New York Times,* April 4, 2020. https://www.nytimes
.com/2020/04/04/us/coronavirus-china-travel-restrictions.html.

Fallows, James. 2020. "The Three Weeks That Changed Everything." *Atlantic,*
June 29, 2020. https://www.theatlantic.com/politics/archive/2020/06/how
-white-house-coronavirus-response-went-wrong/613591/.

Ferguson, Andrew. 2020. "Trump's 5 O'Clock Follies." *Atlantic,* April 25, 2020.
https://www.theatlantic.com/ideas/archive/2020/04/trumps-5-oclock
-follies/610717/.

Fottrell, Quentin. 2020. "Trump Floats Idea of Disinfectant for Coronavirus."
MarketWatch, April 24, 2020. https://www.marketwatch.com/story
/trump-suggests-disinfectant-as-treatment-for-coronavirus-by-injection
-inside-or-almost-a-cleaning-doctors-call-the-idea-dangerous-2020-04
-24?mod=article_inline.

Gandel, Stephen. 2020. "Paycheck Protection Program Billions Went to Large
Companies and Missed Virus Hot Spots." CBS News, April 20, 2020.
https://www.cbsnews.com/news/paycheck-protection-program-small
-businesses-large-companies-coroanvirus/.

Ghitis, Frida. 2020. "Trump Is Fighting a Public Health Crisis with Denial and
Self-Promotion." CNN, May 1, 2020. https://www.cnn.com/2020/05/01
/opinions/trump-coronavirus-denial-and-self-promotion-ghitis/index
.html.

Gilson, Dave, Laura Thompson, and Clara Jeffery. 2020. "Trump's 100 Days of
Deadly Coronavirus Denial." *Mother Jones,* April 29, 2020. https://www
.motherjones.com/politics/2020/04/trump-coronavirus-timeline/.

Graham, David A. 2020. "Why Trump Just Can't Quit His Daily Press Conferences." *Atlantic,* April 27, 2020. https://www.theatlantic.com/ideas/archive
/2020/04/end-trumps-coronavirus-briefing/610771/.

Grisales, Claudia, Kelsey Snell, Susan Davis, and Barbara Sprunt. 2020. "President Trump Signs $2 Trillion Coronavirus Rescue Package into Law."
NPR, March 27, 2020. https://www.npr.org/2020/03/27/822062909
/house-aims-to-send-2-trillion-rescue-package-to-president-to-stem
-coronavirus-cr.

Irwin, Neil. 2020. "Coronavirus Shows the Problem with Trump's Stock Market
Boasting." *New York Times,* February 26, 2020. https://www.nytimes.com
/2020/02/26/upshot/coronavirus-trump-stock-market.html.

Karma, Roge. 2020. "Poll: The Majority of Trump Voters Don't See COVID-19 as
an Important Election Issue." Vox, October 25, 2020. https://www.vox.com

/2020/10/25/21532166/pew-poll-republicans-democrats-coronavirus
-issue-election-economy-polarization.

Kirzinger, Ashley, Audrey Kearney, and Liz Hamel. 2020. "Voters Are Souring on President Trump's Handling of the Coronavirus, with Implications for November." Kaiser Family Foundation, August 17, 2020. https://www.kff .org/policy-watch/voters-are-souring-on-president-trumps-handling-of -coronavirus-with-implications-for-november/.

Kroll, Andy. 2020. "'Absolute Clusterf**k': Inside the Denial and Dysfunction of Trump's Coronavirus Task Force." *Rolling Stone,* April 13, 2020. https:// www.rollingstone.com/politics/politics-features/trump-coronavirus -covid-white-house-testing-kushner-cdc-dysfunction-red-dawn-982308/.

Leonhardt, David. 2020. "A Complete List of Trump's Attempts to Play Down Coronavirus." *New York Times,* March 15, 2020. https://www.nytimes .com/2020/03/15/opinion/trump-coronavirus.html.

Lopez, German. 2020. "Trump's Expert Urged Caution about a Coronavirus Treatment. Trump Hyped It Up Anyway." Vox, March 20, 2020. https:// www.vox.com/policy-and-politics/2020/3/20/21188397/coronavirus -trump-press-briefing-covid-19-anthony-fauci.

Lutz, Eric. 2020. "Trump's May 1 Coronavirus Deadline Is More Wishful Think-ing." *Vanity Fair,* April 15, 2020. https://www.vanityfair.com/news/2020 /04/trump-may-1-coronavirus-deadline-more-wishful-thinking.

Matthews, Dylan. 2020. "Congress's COVID-19 Rescue Plan Was Bigger Than the New Deal. It's about to End." Vox, July 7, 2020. https://www.vox.com /future-perfect/2020/7/7/21308450/extra-600-unemployment-stimulus -expiring-cares-act.

McCaskill, Nolan D., Joanne Kenen, and Adam Cancryn. 2020. "'This Is a Very Bad One': Trump Issues New Guidelines to Stem Coronavirus Spread." Polit-ico, March 16, 2020. https://www.politico.com/news/2020/03/16/trump -recommends-avoiding-gatherings-of-more-than-10-people-132323.

Nazaryan, Alexander. 2020. "How Trump Fumbled the Coronavirus Crisis and Sabotaged His Own Reelection." Yahoo! News, November 9, 2020. https://www.yahoo.com/now/how-trump-fumbled-the-coronavirus -crisis-and-sabotaged-his-own-reelection-190428870.html.

Nichols, Tom. 2020. "With Each Briefing, Trump Is Making Us Worse People." *Atlantic,* April 11, 2020. https://www.theatlantic.com/ideas/archive/2020 /04/each-briefing-trump-making-us-worse-people/609859/.

Nuzzi, Olivia. 2020. "The American People Should See Trump's Coronavirus Briefings in Their Entirety." *New York,* April 26, 2020. https://nymag.com /intelligencer/2020/04/trumps-coronavirus-briefings-should-be-seen-in -full.html.

Oppenheimer, Andres. 2020. "The Way Trump Reopened Economy Will Likely Spur a Second Wave of COVID-19." *Miami Herald,* June 6, 2020. https:// www.miamiherald.com/news/local/news-columns-blogs/andres -oppenheimer/article243331476.html#storylink=cpy.

Pazzanesse, Christina. 2020. "Calculating Possible Fallout of Trump's Dismissal of Face Masks." *Harvard Gazette,* October 27, 2020. https://news.harvard .edu/gazette/story/2020/10/possible-fallout-from-trumps-dismissal-of -face-masks/.

Pesce, Nicole Lyn. 2020. "Three Weeks of Trump Coronavirus Briefings under a Microscope." MarketWatch, April 27, 2020. https://www.marketwatch.com /story/three-weeks-of-trump-coronavirus-briefings-under-a-microscope -2-hours-spent-on-attacks-45-minutes-on-self-congratulation-and-412 -minutes-of-condolences-for-victims-2020-04-27.

Peters, Cameron. 2020. "A Detailed Timeline of All the Ways Trump Failed to Respond to the Coronavirus." Vox, June 8, 2020. https://www.vox.com /2020/6/8/21242003/trump-failed-coronavirus-response.

Phillips, Amber. 2020. "'Totally Unprecedented in Living Memory': Congress's Bipartisanship on Coronavirus Underscores What a Crisis This Is." *Washington Post,* March 26, 2020. https://www.washingtonpost.com /politics/2020/03/26/totally-unprecedented-living-memory-congresss -bipartisanship-coronavirus-underscores-what-crisis-this-is/.

Rothwell, Jonathan, and Christos Makridis. 2020. "Politics Is Wrecking America's Pandemic Response." Brookings Institution, September 17, 2020. https://www.brookings.edu/blog/up-front/2020/09/17/politics-is -wrecking-americas-pandemic-response/.

Saletan, William. 2020. "The Trump Pandemic." *Slate*, August 9, 2020. https:// slate.com/news-and-politics/2020/08/trump-coronavirus-deaths -timeline.html.

Santucci, Jeanine. 2020. "What We Know about the Coronavirus Task Force Now That Mike Pence Is in Charge." *USA Today,* February 27, 2020. https://www.usatoday.com/story/news/politics/2020/02/27/coronavirus -what-we-know-mike-pence-and-task-force/4891905002/.

Schneider, Howard. 2020. "A Quick Reopening, a Surge in Infections, and a U.S. Recovery at Risk." Reuters, June 26, 2020. https://www.reuters.com /article/us-usa-economy-recovery-analysis/a-quick-reopening-a-surge-in -infections-and-a-u-s-recovery-at-risk-idUSKBN23X2CF.

Serwer, Adam. 2020. "The Coronavirus Was an Emergency until Trump Found Out Who Was Dying." *Atlantic,* May 8, 2020. https://www.the atlantic.com/ideas/archive/2020/05/americas-racial-contract-showing /611389/.

Shear, Michael D., Noah Weiland, Eric Lipton, Maggie Haberman, and David E. Sanger. 2020. "Inside Trump's Failure: The Rush to Abandon Leadership Role on the Virus." *New York Times,* July 19, 2020. https://www.nytimes .com/2020/07/18/us/politics/trump-coronavirus-response-failure -leadership.html.

Stolberg, Sheryl Gay, and Noah Weiland. 2020. "Study Finds 'Single Largest Driver' of Coronavirus Misinformation: Trump." *New York Times,* October 22, 2020. https://www.nytimes.com/2020/09/30/us/politics/trump -coronavirus-misinformation.html.

Weber, Peter. 2020. "Trump Wants Praise for His Coronavirus Response. Here It Is." *The Week,* April 25, 2020. https://theweek.com/articles/909198/trump -wants-praise-coronavirus-response-here.

Wilkie, Christina, and Amanda Macias. 2020. "Trump Removes Inspector General Overseeing $2 Trillion Coronavirus Relief Package Days after He Was Appointed." CNBC, April 7, 2020. https://www.cnbc.com/2020/04 /07/coronavirus-relief-trump-removes-inspector-general-overseeing-2 -trillion-package.html.

Yglesias, Matthew. 2020. "Cable News Should Cancel the Trump Show." Vox, March 23, 2020. https://www.vox.com/2020/3/23/21190362/trump-daily -coronavirus-briefing-fox-cnn-msnbc.

State Lockdowns and Reopenings

Alberta, Tim. 2020. "'The Woman in Michigan' Goes National." Politico, April 9, 2020. https://www.politico.com/news/magazine/2020/04/09/gretchen -whitmer-governor-michigan-profile-2020-coronavirus-biden-vp-177791.

Balz, Dan. 2020. "As Washington Stumbled, Governors Stepped to the Forefront." *Washington Post,* May 3, 2020. https://www.washingtonpost.com /graphics/2020/politics/power-to-states-and-governors-during -coronavirus/.

BBC News. 2020. "Coronavirus Lockdown Protests: What's Behind the U.S. Protests?" April 21, 2020. https://www.bbc.com/news/world-us-canada -52359100.

BBC News. 2020. "Coronavirus: Trump Feuds with Governors over Authority." April 14, 2020. https://www.bbc.com/news/world-us-canada-52274969.

Curley, Christopher. 2020. "It's Unlikely the U.S. Will Have Another COVID-19 Lockdown No Matter How High the Numbers Get." Healthline, September 30, 2020. https://www.healthline.com/health-news/its-unlikely-the -us-will-have-another-covid-19-lockdown-no-matter-how-high-the -numbers-get.

Gamio, Lazaro. 2020. "How Coronavirus Cases Have Risen since States Reopened." *New York Times,* July 9, 2020. https://www.nytimes.com/interactive/2020 /07/09/us/coronavirus-cases-reopening-trends.html.

Garcia, Joaquin, Zahavah Levine, Bea Phi, Peter Prindiville, Jeff Rodriguez, Lexi Rubow, and Grace Scullion. 2020. "Wisconsin's 2020 Primary in the Wake of COVID-19." Lawfare, August 10, 2020. https://www.lawfareblog .com/wisconsins-2020-primary-wake-covid-19.

Glanz, James, and Campbell Robertson. 2020. "Lockdown Delays Cost at Least 36,000 Lives, Data Show." *New York Times,* May 20, 2020. https://www .nytimes.com/2020/05/20/us/coronavirus-distancing-deaths.html.

Graham, Bryan Arman. 2020. "'Swastikas and Nooses': Governor Slams 'Racism' of Michigan Lockdown Protest." *Guardian,* May 3, 2020. https://www .theguardian.com/us-news/2020/may/03/michigan-gretchen-whitmer -lockdown-protest-racism.

Hutchinson, Bill. 2020. "'Operation Gridlock': Convoy in Michigan's Capital Protests Stay-at-Home Orders." ABC News, April 1, 2020. https://abcnews.go.com/US/convoy-protesting-stay-home-orders-targets-michigans-capital/story?id=70138816.

Kates, Jennifer, Josh Michaud, and Jennifer Tolbert. 2020. "Stay-at-Home Orders to Fight COVID-19 in the United States: The Risks of a Scattershot Approach." Kaiser Family Foundation, April 5, 2020. https://www.kff.org/coronavirus-policy-watch/stay-at-home-orders-to-fight-covid19/.

Knotts, Brittany, and Meghna Chakrabarti. 2020. "The Role of Governors and the Federal Government during the Coronavirus Pandemic." WBUR, April 16, 2020. https://www.wbur.org/onpoint/2020/04/16/kathleen-sebelius-coronavirus-states-government.

Lopez, German. 2020. "Experts Say COVID-19 Cases Are Likely about to Surge." Vox, October 5, 2020. https://www.vox.com/future-perfect/2020/9/28/21451436/covid-19-coronavirus-pandemic-fall-winter-third-wave.

Maqbool, Aleem. 2020. "Coronavirus: The U.S. Resistance to a Continued Lockdown." BBC News, April 27, 2020. https://www.bbc.com/news/world-us-canada-52417610.

Perkins, Tom. 2020. "'Big Gretch': How the Pandemic Pushed Michigan's Governor into the Spotlight." *Guardian,* May 13, 2020. https://www.theguardian.com/us-news/2020/may/13/gretchen-whitmer-michigan-governor-coronavirus.

Picchi, Aimee. 2020. "Coronavirus Surge in States That Rushed to Reopen Is Hurting Economic Growth." CBS News, June 29, 2020. https://www.cbsnews.com/news/coronavirus-states-rushed-reopen-hurting-economic-growth/.

Reston, Maeve. 2020. "Governors Dispute Trump's Claim that There's Enough Coronavirus Testing." CNN, April 19, 2020. https://www.cnn.com/2020/04/19/politics/trump-governors-coronavirus-testing/index.html.

Root, Danielle. 2020. "Wisconsin Primary Shows Why States Must Prepare Their Elections for the Coronavirus." Center for American Progress, April 27, 2020. https://www.americanprogress.org/issues/democracy/news/2020/04/27/484013/wisconsin-primary-shows-states-must-prepare-elections-coronavirus/.

Rosenhall, Laurel. 2020. "Governor Gavin Newsom Just Slow-Walked California into a Mass Retreat from a Virus. How?" CalMatters, March 20, 2020. https://calmatters.org/politics/2020/03/gavin-newsom-california-coronavirus-shutdown-order/.

Shesgreen, Deirdre, and Maureen Groppe. 2020. "Anti-Quarantine Protests, Trump Pressure Put Governors on Political Tightrope over Coronavirus." *USA Today,* April 22, 2020. https://www.usatoday.com/story/news/world/2020/04/22/coronavirus-governors-michigan-whitmer-florida-desantis-key-states-face-trump-pressure-amid-response/5169260002/.

Smith, Allan. 2020. "Trump Backs Down after Cuomo, Other Governors Unite on Coronavirus Response." NBC News, April 14, 2020. https://www.nbcnews.com/politics/donald-trump/trump-backs-down-after-cuomo-governors-unite-coronavirusk-response-n1183471.

Subramanian, Courtney. 2020. "Trump Accuses Democratic Governors of Keeping Lockdowns Because of 'Politics' as He Visits Michigan." *USA Today,* May 21, 2020. https://www.usatoday.com/story/news/politics/2020/05/21/corona virus-trump-blasts-democrats-over-lockdowns-michigan-visit/5235638002/.

Impact on American Life

Chidambaram, Priya. 2020. "The Implications of COVID-19 for Mental Health and Substance Use." Kaiser Family Foundation, August 21, 2020. https://www.kff.org/coronavirus-covid-19/issue-brief/the-implications-of-covid-19-for-mental-health-and-substance-use/.

Christiani, Leah, Marc J. Hetherington, Michael MacKuen, Graeme Robertson, and Emily Wager. 2020. "To Fight the Coronavirus, Most Americans Support Universal Testing and Mandatory Quarantines." *Washington Post,* May 15, 2020. https://www.washingtonpost.com/politics/2020/05/15/fight-coronavirus-most-americans-support-universal-testing-mandatory-quarantines/.

"The Coronavirus Spring: The Historic Closing of U.S. Schools." 2020. *Education Week,* July 1, 2020. https://www.edweek.org/ew/section/multimedia/the-coronavirus-spring-the-historic-closing-of.html.

Doherty, Carroll. 2020. "Republicans, Democrats Move Even Further Apart in Coronavirus Concerns." Pew Research Center, June 25, 2020. https://www.pewresearch.org/politics/2020/06/25/republicans-democrats-move-even-further-apart-in-coronavirus-concerns/.

Ellison, Katherine. 2020. "Stress from the Pandemic Can Destroy Relationships with Friends—Even Families." *Washington Post,* August 7, 2020. https://www.washingtonpost.com/health/stress-from-the-pandemic-can-destroy-relationships-with-friends—even-families/2020/08/07/d95216f4-d665-11ea-aff6-220dd3a14741_story.html.

"Here's Our List of Colleges' Reopening Models." *Chronicle of Higher Education,* October 1, 2020. https://www.chronicle.com/article/heres-a-list-of-colleges-plans-for-reopening-in-the-fall/.

Hetherington, Marc J., and Isaac D. Mehlhaff. 2020. "American Attitudes toward COVID-19 Are Divided by Party. The Pandemic Itself Might Undo That." *Washington Post,* August 18, 2020. https://www.washingtonpost.com/politics/2020/08/18/american-attitudes-toward-covid-19-are-divided-by-party-pandemic-itself-might-undo-that/.

Jurkowitz, Mark, and Amy Mitchell. 2020. "Cable TV and COVID-19." Pew Research Center, April 1, 2020. https://www.journalism.org/2020/04/01/cable-tv-and-covid-19-how-americans-perceive-the-outbreak-and-view-media-coverage-differ-by-main-news-source/.

Kerr, Emma. 2020. "Why Students Are Seeking Refunds during COVID-19." *U.S. News and World Report,* April 22, 2020. https://www.usnews.com/education/best-colleges/paying-for-college/articles/college-tuition-refunds-discounts-an-uphill-battle-amid-coronavirus?rec-type=sailthru.

Kohli, Sajal, Björn Timelin, Victor Fabius, and Sofia Moulvad Veran. 2020. "How COVID-19 Is Changing Consumer Behavior—Now and Forever." McKinsey and Company, July 30, 2020. https://www.mckinsey.com/~ /media/mckinsey/industries/retail/our%20insights/how%20covid%20 19%20is%20changing%20consumer%20behavior%20now%20 and%20forever/how-covid-19-is-changing-consumer-behaviornow -and-forever.pdf.

Liu, Yi-Ling. 2020. "Is COVID-19 Changing Our Relationships?" BBC Future, June 4, 2020. https://www.bbc.com/future/article/20200601-how-is-covid -19-is-affecting-relationships.

Lukpat, Alyssa. 2020. "Alcohol during the Pandemic: Study Breaks Down Who's Drinking More, and How Much." *Seattle Times,* July 20, 2020. https:// www.seattletimes.com/nation-world/alcohol-during-the-pandemic -study-breaks-down-whos-drinking-more-and-how-much/.

Mozes, Alan. 2020. "Study Finds Rise in Domestic Violence during COVID." WebMD, August 18, 2020. https://www.webmd.com/lung/news/20200818 /radiology-study-suggests-horrifying-rise-in-domestic-violence-during -pandemic#1.

North, Anna. 2020. "We Need to Talk about What School Closures Mean for Kids with Disabilities." Vox, August 6, 2020. https://www.vox.com /2020/8/6/21353154/schools-reopening-covid-19-special-education -disabilities.

NYU Langone. 2020. "A Work in Progress: Family Resilience and COVID-19." https://nyulangone.org/news/work-progress-family-resilience-covid-19.

Parker, Kim. 2020. "Most Americans Say Coronavirus Outbreak Has Impacted Their Lives." Pew Research Center, March 30, 2020. https://www.pew socialtrends.org/2020/03/30/most-americans-say-coronavirus-outbreak -has-impacted-their-lives/.

Parker, Kim, Rachel Minkin, and Jesse Bennett. 2020. "Economic Fallout from COVID-19 Continues to Hit Lower-Income Americans the Hardest." Pew Research Center, September 24, 2020. https://www.pewsocialtrends.org /2020/09/24/economic-fallout-from-covid-19-continues-to-hit-lower -income-americans-the-hardest/.

Parshley, Lois. 2020. "'This Is Exactly What We've Been Warning About': Why Some School Reopenings Have Backfired." Vox, August 17, 2020. https:// www.vox.com/2020/8/17/21371822/covid-19-prevention-kids-georgia -mississippi-texas.

Quintana, Chris. 2020. "COVID-19 Will Hit Colleges When Students Arrive for Fall Semester. So Why Open at All? Money Is a Factor." *USA Today,* August 17, 2020. https://www.usatoday.com/story/news/education/2020 /08/17/covid-cases-college-fall-semester-tuition/5591245002/.

Rosner, Elizabeth. 2020. "U.S. Divorce Rates Skyrocket amid COVID-19 Pandemic." *New York Post,* September 1, 2020. https://nypost.com/2020/09 /01/divorce-rates-skyrocket-in-u-s-amid-covid-19/.

Schleicher, Andreas. 2020. "The Impact of COVID-19 on Education." Organisation for Economic Co-operation and Development, 2020. https://www.oecd .org/education/the-impact-of-covid-19-on-education-insights-education -at-a-glance-2020.pdf.

Schweigershausen, Erica. 2020. "What's Going on with School Reopenings?" *The Cut,* September 29, 2020. https://www.thecut.com/2020/09/will-schools -open-in-the-fall-reopening-statuses-explained.html.

Thomson-DeVeaux, Amelia. 2020. "Republicans and Democrats See COVID-19 Very Differently. Is That Making People Sick?" FiveThirtyEight, July 23, 2020. https://fivethirtyeight.com/features/republicans-and-democrats-see -covid-19-very-differently-is-that-making-people-sick/.

Index

bioterrorism, 12
Birx, Deborah, 51–52, 54, 67, 113–118
black Americans, 86
Black Monday, 45
Black Monday II, 47
black populations, COVID-related
deaths among, 86
Black Thursday, 46
bodily fluids, AIDS transmission
through, 10–11
Bolton, John, 26
Borio, Luciana, 27–28
Bostic, Raphael, 89
Boston, COVID-19 cases in, 58
Boston Marathon, 2020, cancellation
of, 42
Bryan, Bill, 55
bubonic plague, 9, 10
Bush, George W., 75, 115, 126
bushmeat, 10, 13
businesses. *See also* small businesses
aid to, 74
closure, permanent of, 45
closure of, 1
reopening, 66, 70
shutdown of, 29, 43, 59, 60, 62, 72,
83–84, 93, 108

California
COVID-19 cases in, 58, 128
federal assistance sought by
governor of, 63
stay-at-home order issued by, 4,
60–62, 121, 139
carryout food service, 59, 143
CDC. *See* U.S. Centers for Disease
Control and Prevention (CDC)
Center for American Progress, 82
Chao, Elaine, 76
Chicago, COVID-19 cases in, 58
childcare, 4, 83, 93, 99
children
COVID-19 cases among, 102
COVID-19 risk to, 97, 101

of essential workers, 99
from low-income families, 100
SARS-CoV-2 vulnerability of, 58
China
COVID-19 containment within, 34
COVID-19 outbreak reported by,
23, 24
COVID-19 spread outside of, 20, 34
COVID-19 testing in, 66
first COVID-19 cases appearing in,
2, 115, 120, 137
novel coronavirus emergence in,
16–22
SARS outbreak, handling of, 11
China travel to United States
prior to suspension, 27
suspension of, 2, 138
Chinese National Health
Commission, 17–18
Chinese New Year, 19
chloroquine, 54
Choi, Paul, 36
Christmas, 89
chronic health conditions, 95
"circuit breaker" (term), 45
city mayors, 4
classrooms, disinfecting, 102
cleansing products, injecting or
ingesting, 55–56
climate change, 12
Clinton, Bill, 114, 119
Clinton, Hillary, 136
clusters, prevention of, 34
college plans, rethinking, 103
colleges and universities, COVID-19
transmission on, 94
colleges and universities, tuition
income decline at, 103
college students, school closure
impact on, 103
common cold, 11, 105
communicability, understanding, 10
community health measures, 35, 36
community spread, 32, 34, 57

About the Author

Laurie Collier Hillstrom is a freelance writer and editor based in Michigan. She is the author of fifty books in the areas of American history, biography, and current events. Her published works include five previous volumes in the 21st-Century Turning Points series as well as *Alexandria Ocasio-Cortez: A Biography* and *Defining Moments: The Constitution and the Bill of Rights*.